A PATIENT'S GUIDE TO

PCOS

A PATIENT'S GUIDE TO

PCOS

UNDERSTANDING—AND REVERSING— POLYCYSTIC OVARY SYNDROME

WALTER FUTTERWEIT, M.D., F.A.C.P., F.A.C.E.,
WITH GEORGE RYAN

NUTRITION EDITOR
MARTHA MCKITTRICK, R.D., C.D.N., C.D.E.

A LYNN SONBERG BOOK

A Holt Paperback

HENRY HOLT AND COMPANY

NEW YORK

Holt Paperbacks
Henry Holt and Company, LLC
Publishers since 1866
175 Fifth Avenue
New York, New York 10010
www.henryholt.com

Distributed in Canada by H. B. Fenn and Company Ltd.

Library of Congress Cataloging-in-Publication Data

Futterweit, Walter.
    A patient's guide to PCOS : understanding—and reversing—polycystic ovary
    syndrome / Walter Futterweit with George Ryan ; nutrition editor, Martha
    McKittrick.—1st Holt Paperbacks ed.
        p. cm.
    "A Lynn Sonberg book."
    Includes bibliographical references.
    ISBN-13: 978-0-8050-7828-2
    ISBN-10: 0-8050-7828-2
    1. Polycystic ovary syndrome—Popular works.   I. Title: Patient's guide to
    polycystic ovary syndrome.   II. Ryan, George.   III. Title.

    RG480.S7F877 2006
    618.1'1—dc22   2005054748

Henry Holt books are available for special promotions and premiums.
For details contact: Director, Special Markets.

First Edition 2006

Designed by Meryl Sussman Levavi

Printed in the United States of America

10 9 8

To my beloved wife, Gloria, who has always understood my dedication to the art and science of medicine, and who has unselfishly tolerated the endless hours I have spent in my pursuit of knowledge, self-fulfillment, and writing.

To my dear children, Lorelle, Stephen, and Debra, and my grandchildren, Chase, Elliot, Reid, and Spencer, whose loving spirits give me endless joy.

To my parents, Henry and Regina, who afforded me a happy, caring, and loving home.

To my grandmother Frieda, whose love and support during my teen years encouraged me to follow my chosen path to medicine. She was the queen of my formative years, and her spirit and fortitude to this day are part of me.

Contents

FOREWORD

Women with polycystic ovary syndrome (PCOS) can find help—this is the good news that Dr. Futterweit emphasizes from the beginning. Today PCOS is recognized in women as the single most common cause of androgen excess, one of the most frequent causes of infertility, and possibly the most common hormonal abnormality. In the past twenty years, we have also begun to understand the association of PCOS with metabolic abnormalities, including insulin resistance, hyperinsulinemia, and glucose intolerance.

Disorders resembling PCOS have been recognized in women for millennia. Hippocrates, in about 400 B.C., described two cases of women who developed excess hair growth and whose menses ceased. Only in the last century have the ovaries been recognized as the hormonal origin of these symptoms. The term *polycystic ovary* was first used by Drs. Irving Stein and Michael Leventhal in 1935, although other terms had been in use for at least a hundred years. Few can describe the development of PCOS treatment as well as Dr. Futterweit, who has been actively involved in the study of hormonal physiology and hormonal disorders in women for nearly four decades and was an early pioneer in the study of women with PCOS. He has served as a national advocate for the care of affected patients, both in his practice and in his many roles as leader and advisor to patient support groups and professional organizations alike. His textbook *Polycystic Ovarian Disease,* published in 1984, is now a classic of medical literature.

This book will be of immense value to women who have or suspect they have PCOS or some other form of androgen excess. It underscores the need for early recognition, diagnosis, and treatment, as well as the lifestyle changes that are necessary to achieve better health. The book contains a wealth of information on PCOS, including how it is related to obesity, how to navigate it emotionally, and how to follow through with a detailed dietary approach.

We should be grateful to Dr. Futterweit for letting us know where we stand in the evaluation and treatment of this important and pervasive disorder. I hope you benefit from reading it as much as I have.

RICARDO AZZIZ, M.D., M.P.H., M.B.A.
Chair, Dept. of Ob/Gyn, Cedars-Sinai Medical Center
Professor, The David Geffen School of Medicine at UCLA

Introduction: The Face of PCOS

Martine knew that she had an infertility problem. She wanted a baby, she said, but she didn't want twins—and certainly not triplets. She'd heard that fertility treatments often led to more than one baby at a time, and she knew that wasn't for her. "My doctor told me you were the specialist I should see," she said to me.

In her mid-thirties and a vice president at a well-known commercial bank, Martine was direct and to the point in a businesslike way.

"I don't want a high risk for multiple births," she said. "What can you do for me?"

She clearly expected me to write a prescription and she'd be on her way. I knew her doctor well and understood why she had referred Martine to me.

"It's true that a woman taking the popular fertility drug Clomid has a one-in-ten chance of having twins," I said. "But I assume you've been told that I don't run a fertility clinic."

"What can you give me?" she asked.

"It all depends on what's causing your infertility," I replied.

"Doctor, we're both busy people," she said. "I don't have time for a medical investigation. My husband and I want a baby. The problem is mine, not his. Help me."

"Are your periods regular?" I asked.

"I run in the marathon every November," she said. "The rest of the year I train for it—my periods aren't all that regular."

"You don't look like a runner," I commented. She was about fifteen pounds overweight, mostly around the waistline.

"I know." She sighed. "I'm always snacking. When I don't eat, I get dizzy."

Our brief conversation had already been quite revealing. Martine's menstrual cycles were not regular. She was beginning to develop an apple shape, carrying her excess weight in her middle. This is often a sign of insulin resistance, a condition in which greater amounts of insulin than normal are needed to regulate the blood sugar level. Her snacking and dizziness also suggested unstable blood-sugar levels, probably aggravated by a diet rich in carbohydrates.

Martine noticed me examining her hair. It was auburn and cut fairly short, in a style that suited the shape of her face. There was no sign of any thinning scalp hair, which would have been an indicative symptom of PCOS. She shot me an impatient look. Obviously the last thing she expected from a specialist in my field was my apparent interest in her hairstyle!

"When did you last have acne?" I asked, having noticed very faint scar traces on both her cheeks, not quite fully concealed by makeup.

"About a year ago," she said, becoming curious about whatever game I was playing. "You're seeing me at a good time. When I get it, it takes forever to clear up. I think it's all the chocolate I eat."

Contrary to popular myth, chocolate does not cause acne. The cause of persistent acne in adult women is often a higher than normal blood level of male hormones.

"Do you have much unwanted facial and body hair?" I asked next.

"More than most women, I suppose," she answered somewhat defensively. "I use electrolysis to get rid of it."

"One more question. Have you ever heard of polycystic ovary syndrome, often called PCOS?"

She nodded. "I've read a little about it on the Internet."

I told her she had some signs of the condition, but I couldn't be sure she had it until after a physical examination and some lab tests on a blood sample. We discussed PCOS for a while. I explained that she might not always be ovulating when she had periods, something that happens commonly in women with PCOS.

"If PCOS is the cause of your infertility, I may be able to help you," I said.

The lab tests confirmed my suspicions that Martine had PCOS. With lifestyle changes and medication, she was soon pregnant and delivered a healthy baby. I also prescribed remedies for her acne and unwanted hair.

My guess is that Martine's year-round training for the New York City Marathon helped keep her PCOS symptoms from becoming more troublesome. Not all women with PCOS are as fortunate in this respect as Martine. In addition to having more severe symptoms, many never discover what is really wrong with them. Instead, they bounce from doctor to doctor without ever receiving an accurate diagnosis or effective treatment.

If you've done any online research into PCOS, you may well have come across personal accounts that describe experiences very similar to your own. Keep in mind that not everyone who thinks she has PCOS actually does. Other hormonal illnesses can cause very similar symptoms. You can get a proper diagnosis only from a trained professional, ideally from an endocrinologist familiar with PCOS or perhaps from a reproductive endocrinologist, although a number of well-trained gynecologists and internists have the experience to diagnose PCOS. As one of the doctors who is considered to have helped pioneer PCOS diagnosis and the development of effective treatments, I have a personal stake in getting word out to women affected by this sometimes baffling syndrome. I want women to know that once they reach out to seek help in the right place, help is at hand.

If someone were to ask me what I have done with my life as a doctor, I would say that I have devoted more than twenty-five years of it to treating women with PCOS. Today the majority of patients in my New York City practice are women who know or suspect that they have PCOS. In addition to my private practice, I teach, do PCOS-related research at The Mount Sinai Medical Center and School of Medicine, and am active in numerous organizations that spread awareness of the condition. If you don't want to hear about PCOS, don't ask me what I do as a doctor.

As knowledge about PCOS and its treatment has increased, it has been my good fortune to have been involved in important developments and events. Although doctors still have much to learn about this syndrome, we have developed effective treatments for the various symptoms as well as the syndrome itself. The purpose of this book is, very simply, to tell you what these treatments are and how to best take advantage of them.

If you suspect that you have PCOS, the first thing you need to do is make a self-assessment. I help you do this in the first chapter. Take the PCOS Quiz—your score will indicate the likelihood of your having the condition.

Most American women with PCOS have weight problems, and conversely, losing weight can alleviate their PCOS symptoms. A woman's weight may have much to do with insulin resistance. Excess weight and insulin resistance are often accompanied by PCOS, and in chapter 2 we look at the complicated interaction between them.

High LDL ("bad") and low HDL ("good") cholesterol levels, high triglycerides, high blood pressure, and insulin resistance can interact in the *insulin resistance syndrome* (IRS), a condition to which women with PCOS are unfortunately vulnerable. We will look at this syndrome in chapter 3, and at the possible serious health consequences of PCOS in chapter 4, which include diabetes and heart disease.

Part II is titled Getting Well Again, and if you haven't heard this from your doctor, let me be the first to assure you that you can feel good again. The chapters in Part II all focus on managing the symptoms with the best treatments available.

Treating PCOS symptoms often requires the attention of an endocrinologist—a specialist in hormonal medicine, like me. In chapter 5, I show you how to go about find a knowledgeable, experienced specialist and how to establish good communication with her or him so that you can work together to address your most pressing problems quickly and effectively.

Your treatment will work on two levels—you and your doctor will tackle the symptoms that you suffer from, such as infertility or skin and hair symptoms, as well as the underlying condition itself. Let's first consider the underlying condition. You can't cure PCOS, but you can render it almost inactive by losing weight through healthful eating and moderate exercise. In chapter 6, we look at PCOS-friendly foods, namely, foods with a relatively low glycemic index. In chapter 7, Let's Eat, we put those principles into action with healthful meal plans to jumpstart your weight loss. Some of my patients balk at my exercise prescriptions in chapter 8, but there's no need. Even moderate exercise will make a big difference in the way you feel, and the Level 1 plan in chapter 8 is designed for the absolutely sedentary woman. You only move on to more physically demanding routines when you're ready, so your progress is gradual and completely under your control.

Weight loss may be the answer to your fertility problems, because as your weight comes down, so do your insulin levels and, voilà—your menstrual cycles become more regular. But are you ovulating? If you're, not, nothing much can happen. In chapter 9, we show how you can tell. If weight loss doesn't reverse your infertility, we look at two drugs that almost certainly will:

metformin (Glucophage) and clomiphene citrate (Clomid). Separately and in combination, these two fertility drugs have a more than 80 percent rate of success in women with PCOS.

More good news: Women with PCOS can and do have healthy babies. When they get pregnant, however, women with PCOS have greater difficulty staying pregnant than other women. They need to monitor their blood sugar and insulin levels to avoid gestational diabetes. They also need to keep their blood pressure down. If they have previously lost a pregnancy, the drug metformin can help prevent that from happening again, as we see in chapter 10.

Acne is an annoying and highly visible symptom of PCOS. Oral contraceptives usually clear up mild acne; when the problem is more severe, the drug spironolactone is extremely effective. I'll discuss these cures and some simple preventive measures in chapter 11, as well as treatments for unwanted hair and thinning scalp hair. You may need to take these medications for several months before you see the effects, so I'll also cover other ways to deal with facial and body hair in the meantime.

The last chapter deals with the emotional impact of PCOS. Depression and anxiety understandably plague women with the most severe symptoms. As treatment alleviates their symptoms, their mood generally improves, but you can act now to change that, too—many women find help through therapy and/or medication almost immediately.

Finally, I offer a directory of resources available—from online support groups to Web sites that offer accessible descriptions of the latest research—in the hope that this book is only the beginning of your decision to take control of this condition instead of it controlling you.

To see women with PCOS smile again, feel better, be more assured and self-confident, and eventually achieve their goals in life—that must be the aspiration of any physician treating them. I hope this book will contribute to that. It was a labor of love. Readers and patients, I wish you a healthy and happy life.

PART I

UNDERSTANDING PCOS

[I]

What PCOS Can Do to You

A woman usually learns that she has polycystic ovary syndrome (PCOS) because of irregular periods, infertility, or skin and hair problems. Unfortunately she may never learn that PCOS puts her at increased risk for cardiovascular disease and diabetes. Receiving the right medical care can greatly alleviate the symptoms and serious dangers of the condition.

The approximately 6 million American women who have PCOS have ovaries that secrete excessive amounts of male hormones (mostly testosterone) into their blood. A polycystic ovary is one with many cysts—the remains of follicles that never released mature eggs. But polycystic ovaries are a symptom or sign of the problem, not the cause. Three out of four women afflicted with this kind of infertility and other symptoms do not know that PCOS is the cause. Many are misdiagnosed. Some women who come to my office have been suffering from their symptoms for years without a correct diagnosis or proper treatment. This is all the more sad because effective treatments for PCOS symptoms exist and are readily available. Considering the possible diabetic, cardiovascular, and other serious consequences of untreated PCOS, early diagnosis and immediate treatment can be of life-saving importance.

In this chapter, I'll encourage you to take a PCOS quiz and then I'll describe the condition's telltale symptoms. Look at the basic health problems involved in the condition. This should enable you to make a realistic self-assessment of whether to take the next step, which is to find a medical specialist who can make a reliable diagnosis. At the end of this first chapter you should be able to understand and discuss your health problems in a new light.

A DOCTOR'S PERSPECTIVE

You probably have already heard about PCOS and have reasons to think this condition could be responsible for your health or appearance problems. To confirm or deny your suspicions with certainty you will need a medical diagnosis from a specialist, and we discuss that process in chapter 5.

Polycystic ovary syndrome (or polycystic ovarian disease, as it was called until about twenty years ago) was originally named the Stein-Leventhal syndrome, after two Chicago gynecologists at the Michael Reese Hospital, Irving F. Stein and Michael L. Leventhal. In 1935 they published their observations of the presence of large, polycystic ovaries in women with an absence of menstrual cycles, increased body hair growth, and infertility. Portions, or wedges, of ovarian tissues were sometimes surgically removed in what were known as wedge resection biopsies. Women who had such biopsies of both ovaries started to have regular menstrual cycles, and some conceived. This procedure helped regulate the menstrual cycle and enhanced fertility for a year or two, but then irregular periods and infertility problems returned. In the early 1960s the procedure was discontinued.

If you haven't heard much about this syndrome until very

recently, that's most likely because many women and some health professionals may not be familiar with it, not because the condition is rare. Let's start with a few simple questions.

PCOS Quiz

The big question, of course, is whether you have PCOS. You probably have symptoms that lead you to think you might have the condition. This quiz narrows down the really important questions you need to ask yourself. But that is all the quiz does. Even if you answer yes to every one of these questions, this does not guarantee that PCOS is the cause of your symptoms.

The twelve quiz questions focus on three common problem areas.

IRREGULAR MENSTRUAL PERIODS
1. Do you have eight or fewer periods a year?
2. Have you ever gone four months or longer without having a period?
3. Do you have irregular bleeding or spotting?
4. Are you having trouble conceiving?

SKIN AND HAIR PROBLEMS
5. Do you have excessive hair on your face and body?
6. Do you have severe adolescent or persistent adult acne?
7. Do you have thinning scalp hair?
8. Do you have skin tags or velvety, dark skin patches on the nape of your neck?

WEIGHT PROBLEMS
9. Have you recently had a significant weight gain?
10. Do you carry excess weight around your waistline?
11. Do you feel sugar cravings, drowsiness, and sometimes light-headedness within the first few hours after a meal?
12. Do you or any close family members have type 2 diabetes?

Answering yes to five or more of these twelve questions means that you need to seek a diagnosis. If PCOS is not the cause of your problems, something else is. You need professional help.

Answering yes to even one of these questions should alert you to a possible developing health problem. Don't wait in hope that the symptom will disappear in time of its own accord. Perhaps it will, but why wait? It's certainly worth discussing with your doctor.

JANET'S STORY

Janet's health problems began at the age of twelve, with her first period. Throughout her teens, her periods were erratic, occurring only every two or three months, and the bleeding lasting two to three weeks each time. Doctors could find nothing wrong with her. She continually suffered from minor ailments that disappeared in time, only to reappear or be replaced by others. One doctor thought that depression might be the underlying cause of her physical ailments and sent her to a psychiatrist. She developed high cholesterol and weight problems in her late twenties.

Finally a doctor diagnosed Janet with PCOS and explained how it led to erratic periods and unwanted facial hair. Unfortunately the doctor didn't warn her about weight gain and other health problems. At times, she had feelings of uncontrollable hunger. At other times, the smell of some foods could make her vomit. Janet often found that she couldn't stand the presence of certain people, even though they had done nothing to justify her feelings against them and she knew she would feel differently about them again in a few days.

It didn't occur to her for a long time—until she joined a support group—that these problems might be associated with PCOS.

WHAT ARE THE SYMPTOMS?

Polycystic ovary syndrome is *not* a disease in the sense of a single malady, but rather is a combination of various symptoms that share an underlying cause. Some women have only a few symptoms, while others have many. Your symptoms may also vary in degree and intensity.

The following are the most important symptoms to look for. Although symptoms vary from one woman to the next, all women with PCOS experience at least some of these symptoms.

- Irregular periods
- Excessive hair growth on face and body
- Scalp hair thinning
- Acne
- Excess weight, sugar craving, and inability to lose weight (plus abnormal blood lipid levels and a tendency to an apple shape)
- Darkening of skin areas, particularly on the nape of the neck, known as acanthosis nigricans
- Skin tags
- Gray-white breast discharge
- Sleep apnea
- Pelvic pain
- Depression, anxiety, sleep disturbances, and other emotional disorders

You may have blamed these symptoms on your metabolism or assumed (as some of my patients do) that they were a family trait. Some women put up with their symptoms for years, until they decide want a baby and have trouble conceiving. Or they seek professional help when their skin and hair problems become so embarrassing. Other women diligently seek professional help but are repeatedly misdiagnosed.

When I organized and chaired the Polycystic Ovary Syndrome Association (PCOSA) Annual Conference in San Diego in 2000, I was struck by the great number of women there in search of answers and appropriate treatment. Those I spoke to told the same story again and again: They had been suffering from their symptoms for years and—perhaps like you—they were done waiting for help to find them. They were ready to take control.

OVARIES AND EGG CELLS

Understanding how ovaries function in a normal menstrual cycle is essential to understanding what happens in PCOS. The ovaries are among the first organs formed in a developing female fetus. A female fetus twenty weeks old has a whopping 6 to 7 million egg cells. At birth, that number has declined to between 1 and 2 million, and at puberty, a girl has about 300,000 eggs cells. During a woman's reproductive years, about 300 of those egg cells develop into mature eggs. For every one that matures, about 1,000 do not. By menopause, just a few thousand egg cells remain.

When a girl reaches puberty, the sex hormones begin to activate some of her hitherto inactive egg cells. In each menstrual cycle, about twenty eggs in one ovary become activated. Each ripening egg develops in a fluid-filled sac, surrounded by a sheath of support cells collectively called a follicle. Only one of the twenty or so follicles becomes dominant and continues to ripen until the egg is mature, while the other follicles whither. At ovulation, the dominant follicle ruptures and the egg is released and travels through the fallopian tube to the uterus.

The "cysts" of PCOS are dominant follicles that never released their eggs and remain embedded in the ovary. Even when their periods are regular, women with PCOS often have menstrual cycles without ovulation, that is, without the dominant follicle rupturing and releasing its egg. These are called anovulatory cycles.

Why doesn't the dominant follicle release its egg? A higher than normal blood level of male hormones, mostly testosterone, is probably responsible. So what makes the ovaries secrete more male hormones than normal into the bloodstream? Many experts believe a high blood level of insulin is the culprit; in a few pages we will look at other possible causes.

HORMONES AND OVARIES

Let's look briefly at how hormones regulate the menstrual cycle. Some of this will be familiar to you from biology class, but it's probably been a while since you've focused on the details. For egg release or ovulation to occur, a menstrual cycle must take place. The cycle is initiated and regulated by hormone-secreting organs in the brain. The cycle begins with the hypothalamus signaling the pituitary gland to produce follicle-stimulating hormone (FSH), which stimulates growth of the egg follicles as well as estrogen secretion by the ovaries. Blood-borne estrogen travels to the uterus and thickens its lining (endometrium). The rising estrogen blood level signals the pituitary to reduce FSH secretion. This in turn causes the ovaries to secrete less estrogen into the bloodstream. The rising estrogen blood level also causes the pituitary to produce a surge of luteinizing hormone (LH). In a healthy woman, LH causes the dominant follicle to rupture and release its egg. In other words, the woman ovulates.

After ovulation, the ruptured follicle becomes the corpus luteum (yellow body), secreting estrogen and progesterone to build up the uterus lining. If the egg is fertilized, it becomes embedded in this lining.

When the egg is not fertilized, the rising progesterone and estrogen blood levels signal the pituitary to stop secreting LH and FSH. This results in a lowering of the progesterone and estrogen blood levels, which can no longer maintain the uterus lining. The lining is shed in menstruation, marking the end of the cycle.

The reduced FSH blood level causes the hypothalamus to

signal the pituitary to secrete more of this hormone, and the cycle begins again.

A number of problems can prevent adequate hormonal signaling in this complex process. For example, secretion of the hypothalamus must be in a critical range to stimulate the pituitary to secrete FSH and start the menstrual cycle. This can be inhibited by stress and anxiety, eating disorders, and acute weight loss. Other problems can lead to a lack of ovulation (anovulation), few menstrual cycles (oligomenorrhea), or an absence of cycles for many months (amenorrhea).

Research shows that carrying extra pounds can also throw a wrench into the works. Hormone precursors to estrogen may be metabolized in fat cells. This takes place in direct proportion to body weight and is important in the well-known association between obesity and frequent anovulation.

Scientists and practicing clinicians have multiple theories about how polycystic ovaries and the polycystic ovary syndrome originate. That's not surprising when you consider the complex interaction of hormones involved in a normal cycle. Any disruption in the process leading to ovulation may lead to the same result: an ovary that doesn't release an egg. Keeping in mind that PCOS is not a disease but a series of symptoms and signs, it makes sense that different sets of symptoms may indicate different causes.

What Causes PCOS?

Although PCOS is the most common hormonal syndrome in women of reproductive age in the world, there is much controversy about its origin and cause. There may be more than one cause, and this would account for why symptoms vary so widely. Potential causes include almost any defect that can cause excessive male hormone production and consequent (but not invariable) anovulation. Some women may inherit a predisposition to PCOS. If a woman vulnerable to it rapidly gains weight, that may be enough to trigger the syndrome—or make already irksome symptoms more severe.

The following proposed causes of PCOS are generally accepted as the most likely.

1. A defect in the hypothalamus leading to exaggerated LH pulses that stimulate the ovaries to secrete more than normal amounts of male hormones.
2. A defect in the ovarian production of testosterone and other male hormones due to abnormal enzyme action on the pathways leading to testosterone.
3. High insulin levels (hyperinsulinemia) as a result of insulin resistance, which further strengthens the effect of LH on the ovaries (see number 1).
4. Genetic causes: Forty percent of women with PCOS have a sister with PCOS, and 35 percent have a mother with PCOS.

UNDERSTANDING THE SYMPTOMS

We look now at PCOS symptoms in more detail. Hormonal conditions other than PCOS can also cause these symptoms, and such diseases, which are often easy to confuse with PCOS, will be discussed in chapter 5.

IRREGULAR MENSTRUAL PERIODS (FREQUENCY 75 TO 80 PERCENT)

With regular periods a woman sheds the lining of her uterus (endometrium) about once a month. For most women a cycle is twenty-eight days, but a normal cycle can be as short as twenty-one days and as long as thirty-five. An individual woman's cycle is usually of consistent length, unless interrupted. Her menstrual period is also usually consistent in length, from three to six days.

Nearly all women have periods by the age of sixteen. Not

having periods is known as amenorrhea. Pregnancy, overly strict dieting, and major weight loss can temporarily suspend your periods. For example, women with anorexia nervosa do not have periods. By upsetting hormonal process of the menstrual cycle, extreme exercise, high stress levels, or use of corticosteroids and other drugs can have the same effect, as do thyroid, adrenal, and pituitary troubles.

Cycles longer than thirty-five to forty days fall outside the normal range, but before you chalk that up as your first PCOS symptom, you need to consider whether any of the causes just mentioned could be responsible. You also need to take into account that some women have irregular periods as part of their normal physical being. Many adolescents and women nearing menopause have irregular periods. A lot of travel causes this in some women. You need to eliminate as many of these possible causes as you can before looking at PCOS.

That said, they are a characteristic and early symptom—for example, most girls with PCOS have irregular periods within a few years of their first menstrual cycle. Martha, at seventeen, had never had more than four periods a year since reaching puberty at the age of twelve. For the first few years she had thought nothing of it—quite a few of her classmates also had irregular periods. Over time, when her friends became regular but Martha did not, her mother became concerned. Martha was an only child, her mother explained, because of her own irregular periods and difficulties conceiving.

To help your doctor assess your situation, you need to keep careful written records of the dates and durations of your menstrual cycles, as well as any premenstrual symptoms such as bloating, pelvic discomfort, body swelling, and irritability.

Women with PCOS typically have five to nine menstrual cycles a year, with intervals averaging forty to sixty-five days. Menstrual flow usually lasts four to six days. Most women with PCOS have no discomfort prior to or during the early phase of menses. Some women, however, complain of bloating, breast discomfort, mood changes, or lower abdominal distress at that time, and this can vary from cycle to cycle.

Normal twenty-eight-day intervals between menstrual flows may alternate with intervals longer than forty to ninety days. At times, a woman with PCOS may have almost regular cycles for some months.

The fact that her menstrual cycles are regular does not necessarily mean that a woman with PCOS is ovulating. On the other hand, she may ovulate at times and even become pregnant. About one in four women with PCOS have frequent episodes of regular menstrual cycles from the onset of puberty. At one time it was thought that if a woman had regular periods and could conceive, she did not have PCOS. Most specialists today, however, would not exclude the possibility because of regular periods.

You may develop a heavy menstrual flow, sometimes with clots and prolonged bleeding. This is known as dysfunctional uterine bleeding and is more likely to occur in overweight women. Normal bleeding does not include clots and ceases after a few days. Since it can cause anemia or may be a sign of other problems related to PCOS, dysfunctional uterine bleeding requires investigation. In view of the absence of ovulation in most women with this kind of menstrual flow, the uterus's lining may become thickened and predispose them to more serious conditions. Your gynecologist should order an ultrasound study of your pelvis to note the degree of endometrial thickness. Other tests may be required to exclude the possibility that your symptoms aren't signs of hyperplasia, polyps, or the rare possibility of uterine cancer.

The regularity of your menstrual cycle can be greatly improved with diet (see chapters 6 and 7) and exercise (see chapter 8) and with the insulin-sensitizing drug metformin (see chapter 9).

Excessive Hair Growth on Face and Body (Frequency 60 to 80 Percent)

Excessive hair growth, known as hirsutism, is one of three ways in which excessive levels of male hormone affect the hair follicles of women with PCOS. The other two are acne and thinning scalp hair. Any one of these symptoms can be a major blow to a woman's self-image.

Women in some ethnic groups tend to have mild hirsutism, particularly on the upper lip, around the breast areolae, and on the lower abdomen and extremities. In other ethnic groups, women have little tendency to facial or body hair. You may need to take your own ancestry into account before deciding on whether you have excessive hair growth.

When a girl has unwanted facial and body hair prior to the onset of puberty, it strongly indicates that she may have PCOS or an adrenal hormonal disturbance. This indication is further strengthened if the hair growth continues to progress into the mid-teens and beyond. You may wish to ask your mother if she noticed that you had early hair growth and, if so, at what age it began. Rose Ann learned that her mother and her sisters all had what they referred to as "a family problem." Over the years they had worked out various effective ways to get rid of their unwanted hair, but it hadn't occurred to any of them that a medical problem might be involved.

When excessive hair growth is caused by elevated male hormone levels, the hairs are usually somewhat thicker and darker, and grow back rather quickly. This kind of hair growth is especially common on the chin and lower sideburns, the front of the neck under the jaws, the upper back and shoulders, the upper chest, the upper abdomen, the lower back, and in a wide band across the pubic area including the sides and upper area of the thighs. Please note that excessive hair growth can also be caused by an increased response of hair follicles to *normal* levels of male hormones. Oversensitive hair follicles are often genetic. If such hair growth is not accompanied by menstrual irregularities, it does not alone signify that you have PCOS.

Before you blame PCOS for your excessive hair growth, you need to exclude several other medical conditions as possible causes. A sudden, rapid rate of new hair growth can be caused by other hormonal disorders of the adrenal glands, ovaries, or pituitary gland. Some of them are related to benign growths, called adenomas. Your doctor also needs to consider whether drugs are responsible. Such drugs include cortisone-containing drugs, long-term skin application of steroids containing a cortisone derivative, cyclosporine, Accutane, and some earlier oral contraceptives on the market that may promote male hormone-like activity.

A combination of excessive facial and body hair with irregular periods is a strong indicator that you have PCOS. Once you are diagnosed, help is on the way. There are safe techniques to remove unwanted hair, and medications are available to reduce excessive hair growth. I talk about them both in chapter 9.

SCALP HAIR THINNING
(FREQUENCY 40 TO 70 PERCENT)

Hair loss (alopecia) is usually an inherited trait in men and takes place gradually in what is known as male-pattern baldness. This kind of hair loss is rare in women, but can be caused by a male-hormone-producing ovarian or adrenal tumor. As a woman ages she often loses some hair from all over the top of her head. Some women lose a lot of hair after childbirth, but the loss is temporary and the hair thickens, returning to normal in six months to two years. Radiation and chemotherapy can cause temporary baldness. Thyroid disorders and anemia can cause hair thinning. Lupus, alopecia areata, and bacterial infections can cause bald patches. These causes and some others need to be eliminated before your doctor diagnoses PCOS as the cause of your thinning scalp hair.

The following possible causes also need to be considered:

- Genetic predisposition
- Nutritional effects of rapid weight loss or long-term reduced intake of animal fats or essential vitamins and minerals
- Pulling at your hair, sometimes as an unconscious habit (trichotillomania)
- Any tugging force on your hair, such as styling, that can cause hair to be pulled out at the roots
- Cortisone-like medications and topicals, beta blockers (such as Inderal), male-hormone-promoting oral contraceptives, phenothiazines (such as Compazine), and topical chemicals for the scalp
- Dermatitis or psoriasis
- A premature reduction of estrogen production by the ovaries, starting at age thirty-five to forty
- Various medical conditions

By now it's clear you can't assume that you have PCOS simply because you have thinning scalp hair, although in rare instances it appears as the only symptom. Typically, though, it is accompanied by other symptoms, such as excessive facial and body hair or irregular menstrual cycles. Virginia was thirty-two when she first noticed that her scalp hair was thinning. She started noticing unwanted facial and body hair in her teens and could hardly believe the cruel joke that nature was now playing on her. She had hair where she didn't need it and was losing it where she did.

You may first notice male-hormone-related thinning scalp hair as a change in texture. Your hair may become less curly and feel finer to the touch. You may also notice increased hair loss in the shower. Only after you lose 15 to 20 percent of the hair on your head will you see the difference. Much of the hair loss occurs seasonally, in the spring and fall. Although hair loss and regrowth are a normal process, this balance is upset when you begin to lose more than 100 to 150 hairs a day. As you can imagine, there's not much point to counting lost hairs. It will only add to your emotional distress.

Thinning scalp hair due to high male hormone levels tends to be in the midline (vertex) area, and is often first noticed in the frontal hairline extending to the crown area of the head. It appears like a widened hair parting. I have called this the "triangle sign." While there may be some recession of hair above the temples, the hairline remains unbroken (an important sign of PCOS). There is only minimal hair thinning above the ears and upward, unless your hair loss problem has more than one cause. It's a good idea to see a dermatologist, as well as an endocrinologist, for evaluation of this very distressing symptom. I will look at ways to combat thinning scalp hair in chapter 11.

Severe Adolescent or Persistent Adult Acne (Frequency 40 to 60 Percent)

Although acne can occur at any age, you are most likely to have this skin condition when you are going through adolescent hormonal changes. If the acne is severe and resistant to dermatologic treatment, high male hormone levels are often responsible. Menstruation, pregnancy, some oral contraceptives, and other things that upset the balance of male hormones can trigger acne. Girls in their teens often have a flare-up a week before their periods. Acne usually clears in the late teens or early twenties, a little earlier for young men than young women.

The sebaceous glands, which are part of a hair follicle, secrete oil called sebum. This oil works its way upward through the follicle and is released through the skin pore that forms the opening of each follicle. Acne occurs when the pore becomes blocked by an oil plug carrying dead cells and bacteria. If it also contains the pigment melanin, the plug may appear as a blackhead. The plugged follicle swells and ultimately bursts. Having a number of such plugged follicles—usually over the lower third of your face but sometimes on your back or chest—constitutes acne. Increased male hormone levels stimulate oil secretion, which in turns leads to more plugged pores.

As long as the plugged follicles do not become inflamed, the acne remains mild and usually clears without leaving any scars. When acne becomes inflamed, it is often due to bacteria inside the follicle that feed on the oil. They excrete fatty acids that can be an irritant. Normally this is not a problem, because the oil exiting from the skin pore carries the fatty acids with it and they are washed away from the skin surface. When the pore is blocked by a plug, though, the fatty acids can cause the follicle to become inflamed, resulting in a pus-filled cyst. (The use of the word *cyst* here has no connection to the cysts of a polycystic ovary.) On healing, severe cystic acne can leave permanent skin scars.

So many adolescents have *mild* acne as they undergo hormonal changes, it could almost be called a normal skin condition for that time of life. Only when acne is severe or persists beyond the late teens, early to mid-twenties, or even later can it be said to be a likely PCOS symptom. In contrast with the mild form, severe acne is uncommon. Less than one in 100 hormonally normal Caucasian women age eighteen to twenty-one suffers from severe acne. Occasionally girls of age eight or nine who have severe acne and hirsutism are later diagnosed as having PCOS or another male-hormone-related condition. When acne shows signs of becoming inflamed, whatever the cause, I suggest seeking prompt help from your doctor.

Cheryl's friends teased her about being a perpetual teen at the age of twenty-nine! She ignored their ribbing, being fully mature in matters other than her skin. She washed her face frequently with soap and water, used hot compresses, applied astringents to remove excess oil, and avoided touching her face with her fingers. These measures helped prevent the acne pustules from becoming red and inflamed. But they didn't stop new ones from developing. She needed to take additional measures for that, which I'll discuss in chapter 11.

Excess Weight, Sugar Craving, and Inability to Lose Weight (Frequency 55 to 80 Percent)

Being overweight and unable to lose weight is often the main complaint of women with PCOS. They often carry extra pounds around their midsections in what doctors call a central distribution of excess fat. This apple shape is typical of insulin resistance. "I don't want to be shaped like an apple," Kathleen told me. "I try to cut back on food, but when I don't eat, I become nauseated and dizzy. I eat again to make it stop."

Excess weight and insulin resistance are inextricably intertwined. A significant weight gain is frequently associated with worsening PCOS symptoms, insulin resistance, and the insulin resistance syndrome that also puts these women at greater risk for heart disease and diabetes (see chapter 4.) Their desire for sweet foods can become almost compulsive. Sweet, sugary foods are quickly converted to blood sugar and are soon processed in your body. You soon feel hungry again, or even hypoglycemic. High-carbohydrate meals are those most likely to have this effect, particularly those rich in simple sugars, starches, and processed grains. The remedy lies in balancing such meals according to the PCOS Diet Program, in chapter 6.

Acanthosis Nigricans (Frequency 10 Percent of Overweight Women with PCOS)

About one in ten overweight women with PCOS have a subtle darkened skin area that is velvety in appearance and feel. The skin area may also be bumpy, irregular, or raised. Such areas most frequently occur on the nape of the neck, in the armpits, and in skin folds under the breasts or around the pubic area. African-American and Latino women most often have this skin condition. A family member who notices these patches may mistakenly believe that the affected area needs simply needs a proper washing. Some teenagers are ridiculed by their peers. That was more or less what happened to Giselle when she developed acanthosis at the age of twenty-seven. In response, she avoided clothes that revealed the neck area affected and wore a silk scarf.

These darkened skin areas can be lightened significantly through weight loss and treatment to lower insulin levels. Although acanthosis nigricans is a PCOS symptom, having it does not necessarily mean that you have PCOS. Insulin resistant women without PCOS can have this skin condition, as well as some women with benign pituitary adenomas.

Skin Tags

Pale or dark brown skin tags are a sign of excess insulin and imply that the person who has them is insulin resistant. A woman who has them does not necessarily have PCOS, but she is likely to be affected by hyperinsulinemia if she is younger than forty years of age. Skin tags, which are benign growths, are often associated with acanthosis nigricans.

Roni's skin tags appeared in her armpits and on her neck after she turned forty. She clipped off one skin tag with her nail scissors and developed an infection at the site. After that experiment gone awry, she got professional help: Her dermatologist removed them.

Gray-White Breast Discharge (Frequency 8 to 10 Percent)

PCOS can cause a gray-white breast discharge. Such a discharge is also caused by excess secretion of the breast milk hormone prolactin by the pituitary gland. There are other potential causes, with a pituitary disorder at the top of the list. Excess prolactin secretion can also be caused by antianxiety and antipsychotic drugs.

When Allison first noticed her breast discharge, she was delighted because she took it as a sign that she was finally pregnant. Then her doctor gave her the disappointing news. However, the discharge alerted the physician to PCOS as a possible cause of her infertility.

Sleep Apnea (Frequency about 8 Percent)

Sleep apnea is caused by repeated collapse of the pharynx airway during sleep. A sufferer wakes repeatedly throughout the night—that's the body's fail-safe mechanism for restoring normal breathing. Needless to say, it leads to daytime sleepiness as well as lower mental performance and reduced quality of life. It may even lead to high blood pressure, heart attacks, and stroke.

The incidence of sleep apnea is 2 to 4 percent in healthy men and women. It usually is associated with obesity and occurs in many more men than women. Elevated male hormones are also associated with sleep apnea. Overweight women with PCOS who have elevated male hormone levels and a central type of fat distribution have been shown to be four times more likely to suffer from sleep apnea than healthy women. Prudence's friend thought she was trying to be funny when she told them of being repeatedly half-jolted out of sleep. The problem was, of course, much more serious and one that required medical attention. Many believe that insulin resistance is a major cause of the condition. This is supported by the finding of a San Diego physician that one-third of his patients with type 2 diabetes suffered from sleep apnea.

Pelvic Pain (Frequency Unknown)

The frequent presence of pain in the pelvic area, particularly around the ovaries, is one of the symptoms generally not mentioned in medical textbooks or reviews of PCOS. About a quarter of my PCOS patients complain of chronic pelvic discomfort. They may also suffer more acute episodes of sharp pelvic pain, which gradually resolves in a few hours or days.

The pain occasionally follows sex, and Nina wondered if her vigorous lovemaking was responsible. She was relieved to hear that the pain is caused by small ruptures of ovarian cysts, which irritate the pelvic cavity lining. When a major rupture of a cyst occurs, severe bleeding can result, creating a life-threatening situation and a possible need of a blood transfusion. Although such occurrences are rare, their potential for trouble makes the presence of pelvic pain worth mentioning to your physician.

Depression, Anxiety, Sleep Disturbances, and Other Emotional Disorders (Frequency Unknown)

It should come as no surprise that PCOS symptoms can have major emotional consequences. If you are overweight, as so many women with PCOS are, a loss of 5 to 7 percent of your body weight through diet and moderate exercise can alleviate these physical symptoms and consequently ease the emotional distress.

Crystal, at thirty-six, had been diagnosed with PCOS five years previously and found that weight loss greatly relieved her symptoms. But just as things were going well, she invariably became depressed and began compulsively snacking and overeating. Within a month or two, she regained the weight she had lost and her PCOS symptoms returned. She recognized the pattern after the third cycle and told her doctor. The antidepressants prescribed for her helped her keep emotionally stable and maintain a healthy weight.

To date, most published psychological studies of women with PCOS have not adequately addressed the emotional factors in this syndrome. Recently more researchers are undertaking in-depth studies, and I hope their results will suggest fresh ways for women to cope with the emotional challenges of PCOS. In the meantime, it is important to find a specialist who listens atten-tively and sympathetically. This doctor should be someone who can help you have an optimistic frame of mind and assist you on the road to significant improvement.

In my opinion, it is of great importance that the physician treating you asks what is most emotionally disturbing to you about your condition. You are the only one who can say how each symptom emotionally affects you. We will talk more in chapter 5, about finding a doctor, and about managing stress and finding emotional support in chapter 12.

OTHER FACTORS

If any close family members have been diagnosed with PCOS, your chances of having this inheritable condition are greatly in-creased. Because of the role that hormones play in both, PCOS has a surprising relationship to epilepsy. We will look at these as-pects in the following sections. If it turns out that you have PCOS, take heart: There is a lot you can do to relieve its symptoms.

Symptoms in Close Family Members

PCOS often runs in families. As a result, you need to carefully inquire about other women in your family who may have PCOS or symptoms of excess male hormones. How many have weight problems? Do any have excess facial or body hair? Ask about ir-regular periods and infertility. Did your mother ever have ovar-ian surgery or trouble conceiving?

Besides looking for symptoms directly related to PCOS,

you need to inquire also about type 2 diabetes mellitus and the insulin resistance syndrome. Who has high blood pressure or high cholesterol or triglycerides? Who has had a cardiac event or a stroke? Many women with PCOS end up with type 2 diabetes or heart problems. Sometimes these are the symptoms that prompt women to make an appointment with their doctor while the underlying PCOS condition remains undiagnosed.

If there is a family history of PCOS, you are more likely to have it. This applies particularly to a sister, and sometimes to a mother, with a history of many of your symptoms.

On the other hand, if none of the females in your close family have PCOS-like symptoms, you have good reason to wonder why you should be the first and only one with the syndrome. Yet this is frequently the case—or your symptoms may be caused by something else.

Epilepsy's Connection to PCOS

More than a million American women have epilepsy, and the condition itself and antiseizure drugs can affect menstrual cycles. In addition, hormonal changes associated with the menstrual cycle can affect seizures.

Many women have their first epileptic seizures when they begin having periods. As a general rule, estrogen promotes and worsens seizures, whereas progesterone protects women from them. Women are most likely to have seizures just before the beginning of a new menstrual cycle, when their progesterone levels are low, and at ovulation, when their estrogen levels are highest.

Because seizures and antiseizure drugs can disrupt the hormonal signals from the hypothalamus and pituitary to the ovaries, women with epilepsy have an increased risk for irregular periods. This situation is complicated by the fact that epilepsy itself can result from abnormalities in this hormonal pathway. The already complex situation is further complicated by the relation-

ship of epilepsy and PCOS. It seems that epilepsy-related reproductive problems can progress into PCOS.

Women with epilepsy have a 10 to 26 percent higher risk
for PCOS than other women. About 40 percent of women
treated with valproate (Depakote) tablets for epilepsy have polycystic ovaries, and 17 percent have elevated testosterone levels
in the blood despite the absence of polycystic ovaries. Valproate
is the leading antiepilepsy drug that may indirectly lead to
PCOS, particularly in women who tend to gain weight. Studies
of the reversibility of changes are still pending, but it is clear that
changes occur due to valproate.

YOU'RE IN CONTROL

You can't cure PCOS, but you can lessen its intensity to the
point where you're symptom-free. The key is to lower your level
of male hormones. If you are overweight, excess insulin is probably stimulating your ovaries to secrete abnormally high amounts
of male hormones, and thus you need to reduce your insulin
level. The diet and exercise programs in chapters 6, 7, and 8 can
help you lose enough weight to lower your insulin level and become symptom-free.

Some women have trouble accepting that their insulin level
has anything to do with their male hormone level. That's one of
the problems with PCOS—it's a complex condition. Of course,
almost anything to do with hormones is complicated. In fact,
there are aspects of PCOS on which specialists do not wholly
agree. The more you understand the syndrome, the better you
can manage it.

Before treatment, you need a diagnosis that you can believe
in. In chapter 5 we will look at how to go about finding a knowledgeable physician and what lab tests work best in detecting
PCOS.

Then you can take immediate action to relieve infertility, irregular periods, and skin and hair problems by following one of the appropriate treatments in chapter 11. These treatments can ease your symptoms, and you will feel better. But treatments for particular symptoms will not resolve the underlying problem of what is causing them, namely, PCOS. For that, weight loss through diet and physical activity is the best remedy.

Excess weight and insulin resistance are intimately associated with PCOS in many women, and the combination of all three often leads to diabetes, cardiovascular disease, and other serious health disorders. In chapter 2 we will look at how excess weight and insulin resistance affect women with PCOS.

[2]

PCOS and Insulin Resistance

M any women with PCOS are overweight. They are also insulin resistant. PCOS symptoms, excess weight, and insulin resistance interact with one another, making it hard to tell which one is primarily responsible for a particular symptom. In addition, a genetic predisposition for insulin resistance or PCOS may be involved. For example, a woman with an inherited predisposition to insulin resistance may develop it if she becomes overweight and then develops PCOS. Another woman with an inherited predisposition to PCOS may develop it on becoming overweight and insulin resistant.

What we do know for sure is that the great majority of American women with PCOS are overweight and insulin resistant, and they can relieve their PCOS symptoms by losing weight. Put very simply, this is how it works:

Weight loss → Reduced insulin resistance → Lowered insulin blood level → Lessened secretion of male hormones by ovaries

The bottom line is that losing 7 to 10 percent of your body weight through healthful eating—and keeping those ten to twenty pounds off through moderate exercise—can effectively reduce your PCOS symptoms. You can do it.

A PROBLEM WITH BLOOD SUGAR

If you have a weight problem and find it extremely hard to lose any of those extra pounds, you may be insulin resistant. When your organs and tissues lose their sensitivity to insulin, a normal amount of insulin is no longer sufficient to process the blood sugar your cells burn as fuel. In response, cells in your pancreas secrete greater amounts of insulin. As your insulin level rises, your PCOS symptoms worsen. This interaction of excess weight, insulin resistance, and PCOS symptoms is complex and varies from woman to woman.

As a general rule, the heavier a woman is, the more insulin resistant she becomes and the more she suffers from her PCOS symptoms. A high insulin level stimulates your ovaries to secrete more male hormones, and they in turn intensify your PCOS symptoms.

In addition to exacerbating PCOS symptoms by increasing insulin levels, excess weight is associated with two major health problems that affect many women with PCOS, namely, type 2 diabetes and cardiovascular disease. About 70 percent of the Americans who develop type 2 diabetes do so because of increased body weight. In addition, when a person develops type 2 diabetes, excess weight interferes with management and recovery. In the Diabetes Prevention Program study, a 5 to 7 percent weight loss in the first year, with about three hours of brisk walking per week, lessened the development of type 2 diabetes by nearly 60 percent over four years.

Besides slowing the progress of PCOS and diabetes, weight

loss has perhaps more familiar cardiovascular benefits, particularly in lowering blood pressure and blood lipid levels and in reducing arterial inflammation. Only in recent years has it been fully realized that high blood pressure, high blood lipid levels, type 2 diabetes, PCOS, and excess weight can interact among themselves to raise a woman's risk of heart disease and stroke. In chapter 3 we will look at some of the ways in which this can happen in the insulin resistance syndrome. Having insulin resistance does not mean that you have the insulin resistance syndrome. As its name implies, the insulin resistance syndrome is a collection of symptoms that interact with one another as health risk factors.

MARGARET'S STORY

Margaret, a marketing executive for a big electronics firm, sought medical help when she found herself becoming sluggish and gaining weight. Because she had previously been so attractive and lively, people immediately noticed the change in her. Her high triglyceride and low HDL levels caused her family doctor to suspect that she might be insulin resistant, although the result of her fasting glucose test was normal.

Margaret tried to lead a healthier life, but her job required lots of desk work and socializing outside the office. She continued to gain weight and feel sluggish. Then, to her horror, she noticed that her hair was getting thinner. She could hardly count the number of hairs that fell out every time she shampooed, there were so many of them! A dermatologist told her that this trait probably ran in her family and that frequent shampooing would not make the hair loss worse.

Then she saw an endocrinologist. He diagnosed her as having a hypothyroid condition, and Margaret took the drugs he prescribed. When they made little or no difference, Margaret grew frustrated. If she was insulin resistant . . . if her genes were bad . . . if she had an underactive thyroid . . . she could accept all that, so long as she could do something to correct the situation. But so far, nothing her doctors gave her made her feel any better.

She searched around for other medical opinions. What she heard was more bad news. Lab tests now showed that she had impaired glucose tolerance—whatever that meant! She was surprised to learn that insulin resistance is the metabolic disorder basically responsible for type 2 diabetes and that impaired glucose tolerance is a stepping-stone along the way to full-blown diabetes. She also learned that these health problems can be associated with the cluster of other abnormalities known as the insulin resistance syndrome.

One of her physicians discussed her case with me at a medical conference, and I suspected that PCOS might underlie all her troubles. When Margaret came to see me, I found that her male hormone blood levels were much higher than normal, and a pelvic ultrasound revealed that she had typically enlarged polycystic ovaries. Further tests revealed that she had PCOS. When Margaret lost weight and became less sedentary she started to feel better almost immediately. People started to remark on how well she looked. The medications I prescribed prevented further hair loss and helped control some markers of cardiovascular risk.

I explained to Margaret that she was not cured, that she would always have PCOS and would always need to keep its symptoms under control. Keeping her weight at a healthy level lowered both her insulin and male hormone levels, as well as reduced her impaired glucose tolerance. In her case, this was enough to keep her free of symptoms and restore her to her lively, attractive self.

WHAT CAUSES INSULIN RESISTANCE?

Physicians find insulin resistance difficult to diagnose, because it cannot be reliably detected by any convenient test administered in a doctor's office. Although insulin resistance and a high insulin blood level (hyperinsulinemia) usually occur together, doctors often discuss hyperinsulinemia as if it were a separate condition. This is because more symptoms can be traced directly to it than to insulin resistance, and therefore it can be talked about with more certainty.

Many cases of insulin resistance are believed to be genetic, and others may be due to obesity, physical inactivity, aging, stress, drugs (cortisone, thiazide diuretics), pregnancy, and diseases (Cushing's syndrome, growth hormone excess). Being obese triples your risk for insulin resistance, although some obese people are not insulin resistant. Although excess central or visceral fat is typical of people with insulin resistance, many people with an all-over distribution of excess fat are also insulin resistant.

Are you overweight because you are insulin resistant? Or are you insulin resistant because you are overweight? Which came first? The answers may vary from person to person, and each condition affects the other. Discovering which came first is of much lesser importance than finding an effective therapy. You can most certainly do something about being overweight (see chapters 6 and 7).

THE PATH TO INSULIN RESISTANCE AND BEYOND

Eating certain carbohydrate-rich foods significantly boosts your blood sugar level, and any rise in blood sugar is answered by an increased secretion of insulin. Insulin helps your blood sugar enter cells, where it's consumed for energy. Cells store some excess blood sugar for short-term use, and put some in long-term storage as triglycerides in fat cells. People of normal weight don't take in much more food than they can consume as fuel in the form of blood sugar. In other words, they don't ingest many more calories than they can burn.

At some point in their lives, many people begin to notice that they don't burn off extra calories the way they used to. For example, they can't lose weight as easily as they once could. The straightforward balance of calories in and calories burned in a healthy body doesn't seem to apply to their bodies anymore. Often the cause of this is the development of insulin resistance.

With insulin resistance, your body cells become less sensitive to insulin and require more of it to process blood sugar. When this happens, your body detects the presence of unprocessed blood sugar and signals the beta cells of your pancreas to secrete more insulin. Then the larger amount of insulin that builds up processes your blood sugar and its level quickly drops.

A rapid drop in the blood sugar level causes you to feel hungry again and crave sweets and carbohydrate-rich snacks or fruits. You may also have other symptoms of low blood sugar (hypoglycemia), such as light-headedness, sweats, tremors, drowsiness, irritability, or palpitations. When you eat more carbohydrate-rich foods, your blood sugar level rises again. In response to this, more insulin is secreted. You can see where this is going: You're suddenly caught up in unending cycles.

During each cycle, the insulin is depositing some of your excess blood sugar in the form of triglycerides in fat cells. The weight accumulates quickly. The more weight you put on, the more severe your insulin resistance becomes. The more severe your insulin resistance becomes, the more weight you put on. Perhaps through overstimulation, the insulin-secreting cells of the pancreas work progressively less well during prolonged insulin resistance and may become exhausted, leading to clinical type 2 diabetes.

ARE YOU INSULIN RESISTANT?

Here are ten warning signs that you could be insulin resistant. You'll recognize many of these indications from the list of PCOS symptoms in chapter 1, a crossover that illustrates the close relationship between the two conditions.

1. You are middle-aged or older and overweight.
2. You carry most of your excess fat in your midsection, with a waist measurement of 35 inches (88 centimeters) or more.
3. You have acanthosis nigricans (dark skin patches).
4. You have skin tags.
5. You have symptoms of hypoglycemia (such as light-headedness or drowsiness) half an hour to three hours after eating.
6. You have recently gained weight and seem unable to lose it.
7. Your periods are irregular.
8. You have a close family member with PCOS.
9. You have high blood pressure or blood lipid abnormalities.
10. Other close family members have the same symptoms or signs.

Although none of these warning signs is a definite indication of insulin resistance, the more of them that apply to you, the more reason you have to suspect that you could be insulin resistant.

Discovering whether you are insulin resistant may not be easy. The most reliable way to do so is by the hyperinsulinemic-euglycemic clamp technique. This is a complex lab procedure involving infusions of insulin and glucose, and lasting one to three hours. It is used mostly at research centers for special studies.

Regular lab tests performed on blood samples are not as reliable for detecting insulin resistance as they can be for other conditions. Tests based only on a measurement of fasting glucose or insulin levels may be inaccurate, particularly when a woman's basal insulin level is in the normal or high normal range or when her weight is normal. In fact, the presence or absence of insulin resistance is considered to be most difficult to assess in non-obese women with PCOS.

But even if their reliability is often questionable, lab tests—that's tests, plural—are worth taking. It's best not to rely on one test alone. If the results of several different types of tests all point to the same conclusion, you can have more confidence in the verdict.

You will recognize these tests are among those described previously as important for diagnosing PCOS, once more showing the importance of assessing insulin resistance in women with PCOS.

Before taking any of these tests, show your doctor the results of any lab tests you have had in earlier health checkups. Was your triglyceride level high, and your HDL cholesterol level low? This combination of lipid abnormalities is often an indication of an insulin resistance problem.

Although these are separate lab tests, they can all be done from a single blood sample taken in your doctor's office. Therefore, as far as you are concerned, the number of tests performed does not affect you so long as they are covered by your medical insurance, as they most likely will be.

Fasting insulin. Your insulin level can vary from test to test after ten to twelve hours of fasting, but repeated levels of 13 uIU/mL or above indicate a probability of insulin resistance.

Fasting glucose/insulin ratio. This test is based on the ratio between the results of two other lab tests, fasting glucose and fasting insulin. A ratio of less than 4:5 suggests insulin resistance.

2-Hour glucose tolerance test. This test can show that you have impaired glucose tolerance (an intermediate step between insulin resistance and type 2 diabetes, to be discussed in chapter 4), even when your blood glucose level is normal. Two hours after ingesting 75 grams of glucose, a blood glucose level of 140 to 199 mg/dL indicates impaired glucose tolerance. The two-hour insulin levels of people with such results often exceed 80 uIU/mL, signaling increased pancreatic secretion of insulin in response to high blood sugar. During and after this test, such high insulin levels are liable to cause hypoglycemic symptoms. They can be quickly relieved by eating a high-sugar food.

Sex hormone binding globulin (SHBG) test. The SHBG level correlates well with insulin resistance. In women with PCOS (and in most obese women, even if they do not have PCOS), a low SHBG level indicates that excess insulin has caused the liver to make less SHBG, which signifies the probable presence of insulin resistance and causes a high level of free (or unbound) testosterone. The SHBG level is an indirect but important test in determining the presence or absence of insulin resistance. Taking a birth control pill raises your SHBG level significantly, as do some other treatments. In such cases, SHBG is not useful in the initial evaluation of insulin resistance. It can be used as a marker, however, in noting improved insulin resistance with treatment of PCOS. Exercise and weight reduction also improve your SHBG and HDL levels, indicating a lesser effect of insulin and probable improvement in your insulin resistance.

FIRST STEPS

Insulin resistance may be mild to severe, and its intensity often varies according to body weight. You can't cure it, but you can keep it under control. Many people inherit the condition and go through life without knowing they have it or experiencing its effects, simply because they don't become overweight.

Regardless of what diet you choose to follow, losing weight

means ingesting fewer calories. You know that your insulin resistance is improving when your waistline is shrinking. In fact, a smaller waistline can be a more reliable indicator of good control than your weight loss.

As you will learn in chapter 6, high-fiber, high-carbohydrate diets composed of low-calorie foods reduce insulin resistance and body weight. Foods with a low glycemic index do this, too, although some nutritionists claim that the benefits have at least as much to do with high fiber content as low sugar content.

You can also keep track of how your insulin resistance is diminishing by keeping an eye on your low density lipoprotein (LDL or "bad") cholesterol level.

LDL below 100: This is the goal for most people with type 2 diabetes. If you have type 2 diabetes, as many women with PCOS do, your LDL level should be reduced to 80 mg/dL.

LDL 100–129: You have several options. You can increase the intensity of your LDL-lowering therapy and add nicotinic acid and possibly ezetimibe (Zetia) while you intensify control of your fat intake and other risk factors, such as your blood sugar level.

LDL 130 or higher: At this level, most women with PCOS need to combine lifestyle changes with LDL-lowering drugs, usually statins (for example, Lipitor), to reach an LDL below 100 mg/dL.

Another good way to track your progress is to follow your triglyceride and HDL levels, which we'll discuss in chapter 4.

[3]

PCOS AND IRS

If you have PCOS, you are probably insulin resistant, especially if you are overweight. Additionally, you may have the insulin resistance syndrome, in which your insulin resistance interacts with other risk factors to increase your vulnerability to diabetes and heart disease. As mentioned in chapter 2, insulin resistance and the insulin resistance syndrome are two different things. The insulin resistance syndrome—referred to by the perhaps alarmingly familiar initials IRS—is also known as the metabolic syndrome and syndrome X. It can be defined as a cluster of abnormalities and clinical syndromes that are much more likely to occur in people who are insulin resistant. With IRS, such people, as well as being insulin resistant, usually have high blood pressure, a high triglyceride level, and a low HDL level.

Most women with PCOS are insulin resistant *and* have IRS. Because a woman with PCOS is so likely to be insulin resistant and consequently have a high insulin level, the American Association of Clinical Endocrinologists (AACE) recommends that all women with PCOS be evaluated for IRS. Unfortunately this is equivalent to saying that if you have PCOS, you may have a higher risk for heart disease and type 2 diabetes.

I'm not trying to alarm you, but I do want to encourage you to start treatment—including a weight management program—as soon as possible. Cosmetic and fertility problems can cause a lot of suffering, both emotional and physical, but they cannot make you ill or shorten your life span. Heart disease and diabetes can do just that.

In this chapter, we will look at what it means for a woman with PCOS to have IRS. In chapter 4, we will discuss the major health risks involved.

DO YOU HAVE IRS?

Doctors don't all agree on criteria for diagnosing IRS. Some pare the criteria down to the bare essentials; others look for more signs. Taking the former approach, we can say that the following are the four essential criteria of IRS. Having any one, and certainly two, of them is strongly indicative of IRS.

- Triglyceride level of 150 mg/dL or higher
- HDL cholesterol level of less than 50 mg/dL in women (less than 40 in men)
- Blood pressure of 130/85 mmHg or higher
- Insulin resistance and increased tendency toward type 2 diabetes, as evidenced by:
    (i) fasting glucose of 110–125 mg/dL
    (ii) two-hour post-75-gram glucose challenge of 140 to 199 mg/dL (considered to be impaired glucose tolerance)

IRS is a huge health problem for all women, not only for those with PCOS. Your likelihood of having it increases with age:

Age	With IRS
40	33 percent
50	40 percent
60	50 percent

For Americans, ethnicity counts too:

Background	With IRS
African American	36 percent
Caucasian	40 percent
Mexican American	52 percent

Since it's complicated for even the best professionals to accurately assess your insulin sensitivity, my advice is this: If you are twenty or more pounds overweight, you need to assume that you are likely to be insulin resistant and at risk for IRS. If you are of normal weight and know that you have PCOS, you need to make the same assumption and have a glucose tolerance test, blood lipid tests, and inflammatory marker tests (such as C-reactive protein).

TRIGLYCERIDE LEVEL

Women with PCOS often have atherosclerosis-promoting blood lipid abnormalities, among them unhealthy triglyceride levels. Triglycerides, like cholesterol, are a lipoprotein, a combination of lipid and protein. These levels may be caused by insulin resistance or from genetic predisposition, ethnicity, obesity, or lifestyle. Having a high triglyceride level is characteristic of IRS. Your triglyceride level is measured, along with cholesterol levels, in a lab test on a blood sample that you give in a doctor's office. Because your triglyceride level is highly responsive to food intake, be careful to fast for ten to twelve hours before giving your blood sample.

Triglyceride Levels

Very high	500 mg/dL or higher
High	200 to 499 mg/dL
Borderline high	150 to 199 mg/dL
Normal	130 to 150 mg/dL

Fat is stored in the body in the form of triglycerides. Having a high triglyceride level means that you have too many fat particles circulating in your bloodstream and presumably excess fat stored elsewhere in your body, including your liver.

Factors That Raise Your Triglyceride Level

Alcohol in excess
Beta blockers in high doses
Carbohydrate-abundant diet (more than 60 percent of calories)
Corticosteroids
Estrogen
Genetic lipid abnormalities
Nephrotic syndrome
Overweight or obesity
Physical inactivity
Renal failure, chronic
Smoking
Type 2 diabetes

People with IRS who have a high triglyceride level are particularly vulnerable to cardiovascular disease, as are people with a low HDL cholesterol ("good" cholesterol) level. As you already know, a triglyceride/HDL ratio of more than 3 is an indicator that you are insulin resistant and likely to have IRS. These two independent cardiac risk factors, together in IRS, accelerate the atherosclerosis process. These two risk factors can work with a third—small, dense LDL cholesterol particles—to create an even greater threat to the heart. Add to all this the elevating effect that obesity has on the triglyceride levels of women with

PCOS and you start to understand how anxious I am about getting my patients on a sustainable weight loss program immediately.

If your triglyceride level is too high, how can you lower it? Of all the blood lipid levels, your triglyceride level is the most responsive to lifestyle changes. Eat food that is more healthful, lose a few pounds, and exercise or at least be more active and your triglyceride level will probably drop. If you're serious about these lifestyle changes and stick with them, you may not need drugs to reach and maintain a healthy triglyceride level.

- A very high triglyceride level (500 mg/dL or more) requires immediate treatment because of the health threat to your pancreas. You need to eat a very low-fat diet (15 percent or fewer calories from fats), lose weight, exercise, and usually take a fibrate (Tricor) or nicotinic acid.
- A high triglyceride level (200 to 499) usually responds to any diet that lowers LDL cholesterol, along with weight loss and exercise.
- A moderately high triglyceride level (150 to 199) is usually lowered by weight loss and increased physical activity.

Lowering your LDL cholesterol level is the most effective way to bring down your triglyceride level. If your triglyceride level does not respond to lifestyle changes, ask your doctor about medications. Try lifestyle changes first.

HDL AND LDL CHOLESTEROL LEVELS

The problem with lowering your low density lipoprotein (LDL or "bad") cholesterol level is that doing so can also lower your high density lipoprotein (HDL or "good") level. If your HDL is already at a low or borderline low level, this is a valid health concern. It can happen when you reduce the fats in your diet and replace them with carbohydrates, without also reducing your calorie intake. This kind of diet change can lower your HDL level by as much as one-fifth.

Factors That Lower Your HDL Level

Anabolic steroids used by athletes

Beta-blockers

Carbohydrate-abundant diet (more than 60 percent of calories)

Excess weight

Physical inactivity

Fertility drugs

Smoking

High triglyceride level

Type 2 diabetes

Researchers first paid major attention to HDL levels in the Framingham Heart Study. They saw that among study participants with the same LDL level, those with higher HDL levels were less likely to develop cardiovascular disease than those with lower HDL levels. LDL particles, with white blood cells and cellular debris, help build plaque in artery walls. HDL particles help remove such LDL particles from the blood by carrying them to the liver, where they are broken down. You can think of your HDL as functioning like a predator that helps keep the vermin count under control. More specifically, HDL carries antioxidants that probably combat LDL oxidation in plaque buildup.

Women with PCOS, of an average age of only twenty-six, were found to have more of their LDL cholesterol in the form of small dense particles than similar women without PCOS. LDL as small dense particles is regarded as its most dangerous form. Women with PCOS have higher levels of LDL than women without PCOS, independent of weight. They have higher LDL and lower HDL levels than similar women without PCOS up to about the age of forty-five, while after that age, both groups have similar levels. The early prolonged exposure of women with

PCOS to unhealthy blood lipid levels presumably leads to cardiovascular problems.

Cardiovascular Risk and Cholesterol Level
(from the National Cholesterol Education Program)

Total Cholesterol Level	
High risk	240 mg/dL or higher
Borderline high risk	200 to 239
Desirable	Below 200
HDL Cholesterol Level	
Risk factor for heart disease	Below 40
Protects against heart disease	60 or higher
LDL Cholesterol Level	
Very high risk	190 or higher
High risk	160 to 189
Moderately high risk	130 to 159
Mild risk	100 to 129
Optimal	Below 100

The third edition of the National Cholesterol Education Program (NCEP)'s guidelines suggests two main cardiovascular disease prevention strategies:

1. If you are healthy, you can help prevent cardiovascular disease by reducing your intake of saturated fats and cholesterol, increasing your physical activity, and controlling your weight.
2. If you already have cardiovascular disease, you can help prevent further problems by keeping your LDL cholesterol level below 100.

It's debatable which category you fit in if you have PCOS and IRS, and have never had a cardiac event. I suggest that you play it safe by keeping your HDL well above 50 and your LDL between 80 and 100.

Later recommendations from the National Cholesterol Education Program suggest that people at very high risk for cardiovascular disease should aim for an LDL level below 70, and high-risk people who have high triglyceride or low HDL levels should consider combining a fibrate or niacin with their LDL-lowering drug.

HIGH BLOOD PRESSURE

Your heart beats about 100,000 times a day, pumping blood through the 60,000 miles or so of blood vessels in your circulatory system. Each time your heart beats, it builds the pressure needed to drive the blood through the intricate network of vessels. When your blood pressure becomes too high, you have an increased risk for heart disease and stroke. Even moderate rises in pressure greatly increase the risk. For example, in people forty to seventy years old, each 20/10 mmHg rise in blood pressure doubles the risk. The first number of your blood pressure reading is your systolic pressure, measured as your heart contracts, driving blood into your arteries. The second number is your diastolic pressure, measured as your heart relaxes.

Blood Pressure	Cardiovascular Risk Increase
115/75	Normal
135/85	2 times
155/95	4 times
175/105	8 times

As women with PCOS reach age forty-five, they have a higher incidence of high blood pressure (hypertension) than women without PCOS. Typically, women with PCOS have increased daytime systolic pressure. Elevated blood pressure has also been associated with high insulin levels, regardless of weight.

High blood pressure can cause turbulent blood flow. This

turbulence can affect the delicate cells of artery wall linings in the same way that turbulent water damages riverbanks. An injury site on an artery wall attracts white blood cells and clotting factors—the beginning of plaque buildup.

High blood pressure can threaten your cardiovascular health in more complex ways and can interact with other cardiac risk factors. For example, cigarette smoking and high blood pressure are a well known high-risk combination of cardiac risk factors. This combination is even more deadly in people with abnormal lipid levels and among women on oral contraceptives. High blood pressure is also often responsible for worsening diabetic complications, including kidney abnormalities through reduction in blood flow.

Less than half of the 50 million Americans who have high blood pressure have it under control. It seems only half the people on prescription medications for high blood pressure actually take them regularly. To make some changes for the better, the National High Blood Pressure Education Program (NHBPEP) suggests that people starting drug therapy begin with a low-cost diuretic, such as hydrochlorthiazide, instead of a more expensive medication. The program also encourages a renaming of the upper "normal" range of blood pressure to *prehypertension,* in order to serve as a warning. Additionally, you need to be aware that some over-the-counter and prescription medications for other complaints (for example, decongestants) can increase your blood pressure. Ask your doctor for details if you take them.

Blood Pressure	Systolic	Diastolic	Suggested Action
Stage 2 hypertension	160 or higher	100 or higher	Lifestyle changes, plus diuretic, plus other drug
Stage 1 hypertension	140 to 159	90 to 99	Lifestyle changes, plus diuretic
Prehypertension	120 to 139	80 to 89	Lifestyle changes
Normal	Less than 120	Less than 80	

The lifestyle changes needed to lower your blood pressure usually involve weight loss, more exercise, a low-fat diet including more vegetables and fruit, markedly reduced salt intake, no smoking, and no more than moderate alcohol intake.

Salt helps raise blood pressure. Someone with normal blood pressure should not eat more than about 2,400 milligrams of sodium a day (about a heaping teaspoon of salt). Most Americans eat about 4,000 milligrams of sodium a day (about two teaspoons of salt), most of it from processed foods and restaurant meals. That's almost double the recommended intake. Among my patients, those who try not to eat any salt bring their actual intake down to a healthy level—it's hard to eliminate salt completely! Salt is, of course, essential to good health, even when you have high blood pressure, but most of us indulge in too much of this good thing.

Seven Suggestions for High Blood Pressure

1. If you need to, lose some weight.
2. Be active at least half an hour every day.
3. Eat heart-healthy food.
4. Have no more than one alcoholic drink a day.
5. Quit smoking now.
6. Try to manage things that cause you stress.
7. Ask your doctor if any of your medications (decongestants and so forth) might be increasing your blood pressure.

PCOS as Part of IRS

Blood lipid levels and high blood pressure are serious health risk factors that combine with insulin resistance in IRS. Jointly they present a bigger health threat than one of them acting alone. How PCOS interacts with them to further increase the risk of diabetes and heart disease is not fully understood, but we do know they're related. Type 2 diabetes commonly makes the health situation of women with PCOS and IRS even more precarious, because diabetes also interacts with other symptoms and health risks. Impaired glucose tolerance, an intermediate step toward type 2 diabetes, interacts with similar consequences (more on this in the next chapter).

Women with PCOS who understand the real importance of IRS know that as well as combating infertility and hair or skin symptoms, it's essential they take action to protect themselves from diabetes and heart disease. In the next chapter we will look at the major health threats to women with PCOS.

[4]

A Tangled Web

When women meet at PCOS gatherings, they are quickly confronted by one of the great challenges of modern medicine: why apparently similar people in similar circumstances have different health outcomes. True, in having PCOS, they share the same diagnosis. But that's often where the similarity ends.

Your PCOS symptoms are apt to vary according to your genes, age, lifestyle, and medical treatment. It makes you more vulnerable to some very serious illnesses such as diabetes, heart disease, and even cancer, but it does not condemn you to any of them. If you have IRS and PCOS, you're especially susceptible—on the the flip side, controlling IRS is the best way to protect yourself from those other conditions, and you'll lessen your PCOS symptoms in the process. In this chapter we will look briefly at what a woman with PCOS needs to know about diabetes, heart disease, and uterine cancer in order to actively avoid them.

TYPE 2 DIABETES

Type 2 diabetes, also known as adult-onset diabetes, is by far the most common kind of diabetes mellitus. In type 1 diabetes, the pancreas does not secrete insulin and the condition occurs usually in children or young adults of normal weight. In most cases of type 2 diabetes, the beta islet cells of the pancreas initially work normally, but a subsequent decline in their function leads to diabetes. At the time that type 2 diabetes is diagnosed, a number of potentially silent complications often have already occurred, but these can be reduced significantly with appropriate treatment and weight loss management.

FROM INSULIN RESISTANCE TO DIABETES

Many women who know or guess they are insulin resistant have no idea that they are at increased risk for type 2 diabetes. Of the more than 16 million Americans who have type 2 diabetes, at least 90 percent are insulin resistant.

Before you reach the type 2 diabetes stage, you are likely to pass through two prediabetic stages: impaired fasting glucose and impaired glucose tolerance.

I regularly see patients with a fasting glucose of only 90 to 110 mg/dL that a two-hour glucose tolerance test shows to have impaired glucose tolerance. This is an important reason for doctors to do a glucose tolerance test in the initial workup of virtually every patient with PCOS.

With impaired glucose tolerance, your baseline fasting glucose lab test often yields a result of 110 to 125 mg/dL, but you may have a blood glucose level of 140 to 199 mg/dL or even higher after a two-hour glucose tolerance test.

When your fasting blood glucose is 126 mg/dL or more, you most likely have type 2 diabetes, which is confirmed by a two-hour blood glucose level of 200 mg/dL and above with the oral glucose tolerance test.

This progression from insulin resistance to type 2 diabetes can be put as follows.

Insulin Resistance → Impaired Fasting Glucose and/or Impaired Glucose Tolerance → Type 2 Diabetes

Over a six-year follow-up period of women with impaired glucose tolerance, those who also had PCOS were more than five times likely to make the transition to type 2 diabetes.

In the Nurses' Health Study, in which the health of 101,000 women was followed for eight years, women with irregular periods (80–85 percent of them most likely had PCOS) were twice as likely to progress from impaired glucose tolerance to type 2 diabetes as women with regular periods. This occurred regardless of the women's weight.

So if you have PCOS, what's your risk of prediabetes and diabetes? Weight counts. By thirty years of age, obese women with PCOS have a 30 to 40 percent risk for impaired glucose tolerance and later type 2 diabetes. By forty years of age, with no treatment, this risk rises to 45 to 50 percent.

DIABETES AND CARDIOVASCULAR DISEASE

Medical professionals who treat people with diabetes often say that it might not kill you, but it does make you vulnerable to something else that will. Cardiovascular trouble is only one of many such complications. High blood sugar associated with diabetes modifies proteins and further promotes inflammation in coronary and other major arteries. Diabetes also helps produce oxidants that enable LDL to cause inflammatory arterial damage. For these and other reasons, type 2 diabetes is now recognized as an independent risk factor for heart disease and makes diabetic women as likely to have heart disease as men.

To lower their risk of cardiovascular disease, the American

Diabetes Association suggests that people with diabetes older than age forty who have a total cholesterol level of 235 mg/dL or higher (as most do) should seriously consider taking statins and other cholesterol-lowering drugs, sometimes with the addition of ezetimibe (Zetia).

The American Diabetes Association also recommends a target blood pressure level of less than 130/80mmHg. About 70 percent of adult diabetics exceed this level, often because they do not take their medications regularly, suffer from drug interactions, or have difficulty taking drugs. People with diabetes who do not have kidney disease can benefit from most medications to lower high blood pressure. A combination of an angiotensin converting enzyme (ACE) inhibitor and diuretic can be highly effective. While less effective in lowering blood pressure, an angiotensin receptor blocker (ARB) may be the best treatment for those with possibly associated kidney disease.

Unless they have been instructed otherwise, people with diabetes derive cardiovascular benefits from aspirin (which is a blood thinner) taken daily, and/or a 1-gram omega fish oil capsule taken twice daily.

Many women with PCOS develop type 2 diabetes and diabetes-related cardiovascular problems, such as heart attacks and strokes. These major health problems may help to put PCOS-related skin and hair problems into perspective. Of course there's no reason for you to endure either. When you get a reliable diagnosis, you can take charge of both.

PCOS AND CARDIOVASCULAR RISK

Although few specific studies have been made, all evidence points to the conclusion that women with PCOS are at high risk for cardiovascular disease. In the Nurses' Health Study previously mentioned, women with a history of irregular periods (most probably because of PCOS) were found to have twice the risk of developing or dying of a heart attack as women with normal periods.

The AACE called attention to three lines of evidence in a position paper in 2004, of which I was one of the authors.

1. If you have PCOS, you are at a substantially higher risk for developing a combination of impaired glucose tolerance, type 2 diabetes, and serious heart problems. The AACE recommends that all women with PCOS be screened for diabetes as early as possible.
2. Women with PCOS frequently have cardiac risk factors of various kinds (such as blood lipid abnormalities, elevated inflammatory markers, and high blood pressure), and often several simultaneously. These multiple risk factors are regularly diagnosed as IRS, and are associated with an increase in visceral fat (central obesity or apple shape).
3. Imaging studies have revealed that women with PCOS are more likely to have anatomic and functional abnormalities related to cardiovascular problems than similar women of the same age. These include coronary calcifications and carotid artery arteriosclerosis.

PREVENTING DIABETES AND HEART DISEASE

The first steps in preventing these serious conditions is recognizing you have PCOS and getting proper treatment. If you have PCOS, you need to always keep in mind that you run a high risk for developing type 2 diabetes and cardiovascular disease. In this regard, you need to carefully watch out for two things: (1) IRS; (2) silent cardiovascular disease. Diabetic women with PCOS cannot rely on the heart-protective effects of estrogen before menopause. You can reverse some of the risk with early diagnosis and treatment. Your lifestyle should include weight loss and exercise, avoidance of tobacco, and correction of lipid abnormalities and high blood pressure. In the second part of this book, we go into the details of what you can do to protect your health, feel better, and enjoy life to the fullest.

UTERINE CANCER AND HYPERPLASIA

Women with PCOS are several times more likely than other women to develop uterine cancer, caused by high male hormone levels that result in a lack of ovulation. Lack of ovulation in turn results in a lack of shedding of the uterus lining in regular periods. The uterus lining thickens as a result, a condition known as hyperplasia.

Uterine cancer, also called endometrial carcinoma, is the most common female reproductive system cancer in American women. It affected 34,000 women in 1996. This cancer of the uterine lining is most often associated with obesity, as well as high blood pressure, type 2 diabetes, and not having been pregnant. Not ovulating most of the time (anovulatory cycles), as is typical in PCOS, leads to unopposed effects of estrogen on the endometrium, which can lead to endometrial hyperplasia, a precursor to cancer. Although a relatively small number of women develop uterine cancer, you should take preventive measures to minimize the risk. An early diagnosis of PCOS and treatment to end prolonged intervals between menstrual cycles are major preventive steps. Prolonged absence of menstrual cycles is a major symptom and risk factor for uterine cancer in women with PCOS. Drugs known as progestational agents can trigger shedding of the endometrial lining of the uterus. Periodic use of these drugs may reduce this complication significantly.

A Mayo Clinic study revealed a threefold higher incidence of uterine cancer in anovulatory women, many of whom probably had PCOS. A study by the Centers for Disease Control and Prevention reported a fivefold increased incidence of uterine cancer in women with PCOS. Although typically occurring in women approaching or after menopause, uterine cancer or hyperplasia can occur in younger women, even some in their teens. Almost all younger women with uterine cancer have PCOS. The good news is that in younger women with PCOS, this kind of cancer is relatively benign and has a good prognosis.

For women with PCOS who have uterine cancer, treatment is commonly successful after an outpatient surgical procedure called dilatation and curettage (D & C), followed by high-dose progesterone therapy. Younger women often do not need a hysterectomy. Follow-up evaluation by a gynecologic oncologist should include periodic biopsies of the uterine lining. If progesterone treatment cannot reverse the uterine cancer, a hysterectomy may be necessary.

Treatment with insulin-sensitizing agents (such as metformin), oral contraceptives, and weight loss minimize the risk of uterine cancer in women with PCOS. The encouraging data on oral contraceptive use in normal women also show that it decreases the risk of uterine cancer by 50 percent.

As I hope I've made clear throughout Part I, my aim is not to alarm you with the associated risks of PCOS, but to drive home the importance of taking control. The fact that you're reading this book and educating yourself about PCOS is an important first step. In Part II I'll discuss what you can start doing for yourself today, beginning with finding a doctor who can be your guide.

PART II

GETTING WELL AGAIN

[5]

Getting a Diagnosis

We know that excess male hormones, secreted mostly by the ovaries, cause PCOS symptoms. Every woman has both female and male hormones, and her health and well-being depend on the balance between them. When the level of male hormones exceeds the normal range, a woman begins to have physical and emotional problems. This happens in PCOS, but PCOS is not the only condition that causes such problems. Several other hormonal conditions can easily be confused with PCOS because of similar symptoms.

Obviously, when misdiagnosed or not diagnosed for some other reason, your PCOS continues more or less untreated. The best way to avoid such a situation is by finding the right doctor and having the right diagnostic tests performed.

FINDING A DOCTOR

If you think you may have PCOS, you need to find a knowledgeable physician whose diagnosis you can trust. A PCOS diagnosis
is not easy to make, particularly for a doctor who does not spe-
cialize in hormonal medicine. As you already know, PCOS is a
collection of signs and symptoms, any one of which could be
caused by other disorders. For example, the symptom that most
strongly suggests the presence of PCOS is irregular periods—
something that can also be caused by frequent intense exercise
without any associated serious medical disorder at all. There is
no single symptom that can pinpoint PCOS as the cause of your
health problems.

Because of the potentially serious diabetic and cardiovascular risks of most women with PCOS, you need to find a clinical
endocrinologist to make a diagnosis. Although skin and hair
problems may be making your life difficult, preventing the possible development of diabetes and heart disease later in life is
what makes finding a diagnosis urgent. Finding a remedy for
your irregular periods or for your skin and hair problems is not
the same as finding a remedy for PCOS, because irregular periods and skin and hair problems are a result of PCOS, not its
cause. When you discover and treat the underlying cause, annoying symptoms can almost miraculously diminish and sometimes can disappear altogether.

Ask your regular or family doctor or other health professionals for a referral to an endocrinologist. You can research an
endocrinologist's background and credentials by calling the referral service of a university-affiliated hospital or organizations
involved with endocrinology (see Resources). The Internet may
have information on an endocrinologist's position and papers
published in the PCOS field. If you happen to know of a local
endocrinologist who is knowledgeable about PCOS, ask your
doctor to refer you to that physician.

MAKING AN APPOINTMENT

Almost inevitably, the endocrinologist will require blood samples for lab tests. It's best to have your blood drawn in the morning, because later in the day your hormone levels are likely to be increasingly variable, due to normal hormonal changes. You need to fast for ten to twelve hours before giving a sample, so giving a blood sample in the morning means that you can sleep during much of the fasting period.

Try to schedule your appointment during days four through nine of your menstrual cycle (day one is the first day of bleeding) if your menstrual cycle is not highly irregular.

MEETING THE ENDOCRINOLOGIST

The endocrinologist usually begins with detailed questioning about your current symptoms and medical history, including prior illnesses and treatments, and your family history. At this time, or prior to the appointment, give the doctor any earlier lab test results or other data that you have from visits to physicians, even if you think they may not be relevant. In particular, bring any actual films of ultrasound or other imaging examinations that you have had done previously for whatever reason.

In the physical examination that follows, the doctor evaluates the extent of any acne and abnormal hair growth, the degree and distribution of hair loss, and the textures of your scalp hair and skin. The distribution and degree of excessive hair are usually plotted on a diagram, which is later used for reference in evaluating the results of treatment. The doctor also checks for the presence of acanthosis nigricans and skin tags, particularly on your neck. Some consultants use digital photography as a baseline assessment of the degree of skin changes of the acne, hirsutism, and scalp hair loss.

Routine measurements include those of your height, weight, blood pressure, and the ratio of your abdominal circumference to your hip circumference. The latter, also called the hip-to-waist ratio, is an important measure of the central distribution of body fat. Centrally distributed or visceral fat is associated with more health problems than an all-over generalized fat distribution, though this is not to underplay the risks of any kind of excess weight. A hip-to-waist ratio greater than 0.8 indicates a central distribution of fat associated with insulin resistance and probable development of the insulin resistance syndrome. Measurements of 0.80 to 0.845 may represent a potential risk for diabetes and other complications. When the hip-to-waist ratio exceeds 0.85, it should be regarded as a health warning.

JESSICA'S STORY

Jessica had always been a happy child, excelling in both sports and schoolwork. When her periods began, she had very painful cramps. To help with the pain, her doctor put her on an oral contraceptive. As months passed, Jessica had worsening depressive moods. The four doctors her parents took her to all suggested antidepressants. None questioned whether she might be reacting to the contraceptive pill. Her parents took her off the pill, and Jessica's depression vanished.

Within two months, however, she began to gain weight rapidly, lose hair from her scalp, and grow extensive body hair. In spite of exercise, she gained ten pounds in a single week. The doctors thought stress might be responsible.

Jessica's parents desperately searched for information. They had never heard of PCOS, but the writings of a doctor on women's hormonal problems seemed to describe some of the symptoms that their daughter was suffering from. Although they lived in Southern California and the doctor's office was in Ari-

zona, they made an appointment for a diagnostic examination
for Jessica. From Jessica's history and lab tests, the doctor diagnosed her with PCOS. Her mother felt deep relief that at least
now she knew what illness her daughter had and that something
could be done about it.

At this writing, Jessica is sixteen. Seven months after her diagnosis, she is feeling much better and is taking spironolactone,
metformin, and a different oral contraceptive. After five months
on metformin, her body has begun returning to its former shape.
Jessica still has bad days, and her mother regards her recovery as
"a work in progress."

Her mother praises the Polycystic Ovarian Syndrome Association (at http://www.pcosupport.org) for valuable emotional
support. Her advice to parents of teens with PCOS is to take action; find a doctor who can help; keep a detailed history of your
daughter's health; believe in your judgment as a parent. You can
find help. Don't give up.

FACTORS OFTEN IMPORTANT IN DIAGNOSIS

Age
Weight
Ethnicity
Family medical history (PCOS, diabetes, hirsutism, alopecia, cardio-
    vascular problems, blood lipid abnormalities, high blood pressure)
Oral contraceptive use, present or past
Rapid weight change, recent or past, and its relationship to symp-
    toms
Polycystic ovaries on sonograms of the pelvis

DIAGNOSTIC CRITERIA

An endocrinologist considering whether you have PCOS bases
the final decision on a number of factors. The following three
factors are regarded by many endocrinologists as the most significant.

1. **History of irregular periods** and lack of ovulation, with onset at puberty. These signs are often associated with abnormal skin changes, and as excessive hair growth. However, it is possible that almost one in four women with PCOS actually has regular periods, without ovulation necessarily taking place. The symptoms that your primary doctor is most likely to notice are your skin and hair problems. It may be these that cause an inquiry about the regularity of your periods.

2. **Lab tests** that show elevated levels of male hormones. These include total and free testosterone, as well as other ovarian and adrenal male hormone levels. They also include evidence of an abnormal ratio of luteinizing hormone (LH) to follicle-stimulating hormone (FSH), which occurs in two out of three women with PCOS. However, oral contraceptives can change any of these levels.

3. **Exclusion of other hormonal disorders** as causes of the symptoms. Before diagnosing PCOS, an endocrinologist needs to eliminate the possibility that the following disorders, which often have similar symptoms, may be present: adult-onset or congenital adrenal hyperplasia, hyperprolactinemia, adrenal or ovarian hormone-producing adenomas, hyperthecosis, hirsutism from unknown causes, and Cushing's syndrome. We will talk more about these disorders later in this chapter.

We will now look at these three diagnostic criteria in more detail.

Irregular Periods

A history of irregular periods is the first and most significant criterion of PCOS diagnosis. Most women later diagnosed with PCOS experience a normal onset of puberty and menstrual cycles at twelve to thirteen years of age. Some who are overweight or obese as girls have an earlier onset of menstrual cycles. Like those of the majority of young girls, their periods for the first couple of years are often somewhat irregular and are usually painless. As they grow into their mid-teens, their periods continue to be infrequent (oligomenorrhea), but not always painless. They may have two successive periods on time and then not have another for two to six months or longer. They often have no typical symptoms of an approaching period: no bloating, breast tenderness, or pelvic discomfort in the few days before bleeding.

A gradual increase of weight, and particularly a rapid weight gain, may result in intervals of three to six months or longer between periods. An interval of greater than four to six months is called amenorrhea and requires medical attention, regardless of a teenager's weight. One obvious explanation of a lack of periods that must always be excluded is that the young woman has become pregnant.

Some young women have prolonged episodes of bleeding (dysfunctional bleeding), lasting more than six or seven days, and this should be investigated. These bleeding episodes can result from thickening of the endometrium, which is almost continually bombarded by estrogens from the ovaries, adrenal glands, and peripheral stores of body fat cells in a woman who is not ovulating. An ultrasound of the pelvis, with careful attention to the uterus, may show endometrial thickening, which can be measured accurately by the ultrasonographer. At times, there may be ultrasound evidence of polyp formation or other abnormalities. An iodine study of the endometrium (hysterogram) or perhaps a diagnostic biopsy or scraping by the gynecologist may be needed for evaluation of the abnormal bleeding.

IMAGING TESTS

Polycystic ovaries are detected by ultrasound in 90 percent of women with PCOS who have not recently taken oral contraceptives or similar medications. In sonograms of such women, the

ovaries may be normal in size or enlarged, and ten to twelve follicles or cysts, measuring 4 to 9 millimeters, are frequently seen
under the ovarian capsule. Imaging of a polycystic ovary would
seem to be good evidence of PCOS, except that almost one in
four apparently asymptomatic healthy women also have some
features of polycystic ovaries on their sonograms. From this, we
know it is possible for you to have polycystic ovaries without
PCOS. Ultrasound studies of the ovaries alone are not sufficient
for a diagnosis of PCOS, and need to be backed by a history of
irregular periods and evidence of an oversecretion of male hormones, which are far more reliable diagnostic indicators. In addition, other hormonal disorders can result in very similar
sonograms. These disorders include congenital and adult-onset
adrenal hyperplasia, hyperprolactinemia, Cushing's syndrome,
and some cases of hypothalamic amenorrhea.

Although ultrasound sonograms cannot diagnose PCOS
with any certainty, they provide a valuable pretreatment picture
of the ovaries. Your doctor can later judge how well treatment is
working by comparing before and after sonograms for ovarian
size, follicle number, endometrium, and cysts or other growths
(up to 10 percent of women with PCOS develop them). Early
recognition helps avoid the loss of an ovary if a cyst enlarges rapidly. The endometrium can be assessed for thickness and other
changes that can play a role in infertility or episodes of heavy
menstrual bleeding. A thickened endometrium suggests excess
stimulation by estrogen and a potential for endometrial hyperplasia and carcinoma.

Sonograms can even show that you've ovulated in a particular menstrual cycle. The sonographer can see a corpus luteum
cyst—the remains of the bust follicle that recently released an egg.

An experienced ultrasonographer can test young girls with
the scanning device placed against the abdomen (a transab-
dominal sonogram), but for post-teens a transvaginal sonogram
provides a more accurate picture. The best time to have an ultra-

sound is on days 4 to 8 of a menstrual cycle—whether it's a regular cycle or one induced with progesterone.

LAB TESTS THAT SCREEN FOR PCOS

Although lab tests that show elevated levels of male hormones are the second of three criteria for PCOS diagnosis, there is no agreement among professionals on which male hormone lab tests work best. The following are the tests most frequently ordered by endocrinologists. They serve to confirm a PCOS diagnosis, and also to evaluate your glucose intolerance and cardiac risks.

Many of my patients are surprised at the number of lab tests required at my initial evaluation. Not to worry—it only takes one relatively painless stick and six to eight small tubes of blood for a thorough evaluation. Your blood samples should be drawn in the morning, while your are fasting, and if possible during days 4 to 9 of your menstrual cycle. Your doctor could miss early morning spikes in the levels of male hormones, prolactin, and adrenal hormones if your blood is drawn later in the day.

Your lab test results may vary with the regularity or irregularity of your menstrual cycles. Individual responses to hormones vary also. For example, hormone receptors can become sensitized, so that a lower level of male hormones produces the same effect as the higher level once did. The sebaceous glands in hair follicles can become sensitized in much the same way, sometimes resulting in excess body hair even when male hormone levels are at or close to normal.

Testosterone level. Most endocrinologists agree that measurements of total and free testosterone levels are vital in the evaluation of PCOS. Several measurements may be needed of total and free testosterone, or a free androgen index performed by a competent laboratory. Value ranges differ with laboratories, but your doctor is familiar with the lab processing your test. If you take oral contraceptives or other medications, your testosterone level may be difficult to assess.

Most of your testosterone comes from your ovaries, with much smaller amounts coming from your adrenal glands. Free or unbound testosterone, which is only a small fraction of total testosterone, affects the sebaceous glands inside hair follicles, causing cystic acne, hirsutism, and thinning of scalp hair. You can have a normal total testosterone level while having a high level of free testosterone. Much depends on genetic factors, ethnicity, body weight, and individual responses and sensitivity to the male hormones produced. Your total testosterone level is often a good indicator of your male hormone levels. Most women with PCOS have a total testosterone level above 60 to 70 ng/dL, depending on the laboratory used and its normal range. This may in part be due to effects of insulin on the sex hormone binding globulin (SHBG), which dictates the amount of free testosterone measured in the blood. Women with male hormone secreting tumors, HAIRAN syndrome, or hyperthecosis (see section in this chapter called Exclusion of Hormonal Disorders Similar to PCOS) may have varying total testosterone levels of 70 to 150 ng/dL or higher.

Luteinizing hormone (LH) and follicle-stimulating hormone (FSH) levels. An LH/FSH ratio greater than 2 is found in 60 to 70 percent of women with PCOS, and is more likely to occur in women who are not obese. If you take oral contraceptives or a similar medication, your LH and FSH levels will be difficult to assess because the hormones in contraceptives suppress them.

Sex hormone binding globulin (SHBG) level. Women who are obese or have the insulin resistance syndrome also have reduced SHBG levels. Reduced SHBG levels result from excessive insulin production and lead to an increase in free testosterone, which in turn causes many of the symptoms of PCOS.

Prolactin level. An elevated prolactin level may be present in 10 to 20 percent of women with PCOS. About one in three of these women have an associated milky breast discharge and other signs of PCOS.

Dehydroepiandrosterone sulfate (DHEAS) level. DHEAS and other male hormones (androgens) such as androstenedione are weaker than free testosterone, but they are good makers of increased adrenal male hormone production. (DHEAS comes almost exclusively from the adrenal glands.) In initial assessments, most women with PCOS have elevated levels of total testosterone, free testosterone, androstenedione, and/or DHEAS.

17-alpha-Hydroxyprogesterone (17-OHP) level. Doctors test for this female hormone to exclude the possibility that overactive adrenal glands are at the root of the problem (congenital and adult-onset adrenal hyperplasia).

Lipid profile. Your HDL ("good") and LDL ("bad") cholesterol levels and particularly your triglyceride level are good indicators of insulin resistance. In addition, they are a good measure of your risks for diabetes and cardiovascular disease.

Glucose level. A fasting morning glucose level is a guide to your blood sugar status: normal, impaired glucose tolerance, or a clear case of diabetes. Although it is more convenient, this test is not as reliable as the two-hour glucose tolerance test described below.

Insulin level. Because of the technical difficulties involved, this test often has unreliable results. Additionally, a test result showing an elevated insulin level does not always mean you are insulin resistant or have the insulin resistance syndrome. Similarly, having a normal insulin level does not exclude the possibility of having insulin resistance.

Measuring your insulin level, however, is an important part of your evaluation. A persistently high insulin level often indicates a need for the pancreas to release more insulin due to a defect or inability of organs to respond normally to this hormone (insulin resistance). If your insulin level is high or if you have a family history of diabetes, you should definitely have a two-hour glucose tolerance test.

Two-hour glucose tolerance test. For this test, your glucose and insulin levels are measured prior to consuming a 75-gram glucose drink and again two hours later. If you have any symptoms of hypoglycemia (such as nausea or dizziness) during this test, be sure to tell your doctor. Consider carefully if these symptoms are similar to episodes you may have experienced after eating a carbohydrate-rich meal. A similarity between them suggests that you may have hyperinsulinism leading to episodes of low blood glucose levels.

This glucose tolerance test is recommended as a screen for diabetes for all women suspected of PCOS, even those in their teens, regardless of their weight. Since type 2 diabetes evolves over time, any woman who has passed the screening glucose tolerance test needs to be retested periodically over her lifetime.

Other diagnostic tests. Routine thyroid function tests include 1-thyroxine (T4) and thyroid-stimulating hormone (TSH). If your doctor suspects overactive adrenal glands, you may require a cortisol suppression test or an adrenal stimulation test employing adrenocorticotropic hormone (ACTH). A complete blood count, electrolytes, and kidney and liver function should be included in your evaluation. Tests checking for potential risk factors often include homocysteine and C-reactive protein blood levels, as well as a urine microalbumin level.

Exclusion of Hormonal Disorders Similar to PCOS

The third of the diagnostic criteria for PCOS is the exclusion of other hormonal disorders that can produce symptoms and signs similar to those of PCOS. Such disorders do not occur nearly as frequently as PCOS. Of women who appear to have PCOS, 10 to 15 percent of them turn out instead to have one of the following disorders.

An experienced physician excludes these relatively infrequent hormonal disorders through a careful analysis of your medical history, a physical examination, lab tests, and imaging. Treatments for the following disorders can vary dramatically from those for PCOS.

Congenital and adult-onset adrenal hyperplasia. Congenital adrenal hyperplasia, a hormonal condition of the adrenal glands, can cause symptoms that look very similar to those of PCOS. Hyperplasia involves an increased growth of normal cells that enlarge but maintain the shape of the original organ. Although it is relatively uncommon, this disorder runs in some Ashkenazi Jewish, Eskimo, and Hispanic families. The adult-onset type of the disorder can be initially diagnosed by a suspiciously high blood level of 17-alpha-Hydroxyprogesterone (17-OHP), together with an increase in testosterone level. If you have a menstrual cycle that appears to be ovulatory, you not only have an associated rise in serum progesterone, but also of 17-OHP, in the second (luteal) phase of your cycle. Thus it is necessary to measure this hormone in the early or follicular stage of the menstrual cycle—or at any time, if you have infrequent cycles. A diagnosis of congenital adrenal hyperplasia is confirmed by a marked increase of 17-OHP following a safe, one-hour morning intravenous ACTH-stimulation test (Cortrosyn test) in your endocrinologist's office.

Ovarian hyperthecosis. On ultrasound, the ovaries of women with this condition usually look thick and lack the follicles found under the ovarian capsule in women with PCOS (see the Imaging Tests section earlier in this chapter). Women with ovarian hyperthecosis often have significant insulin resistance and high testosterone levels. Many are diabetic and obese, and some may even be fertile. Some experts in this field consider this to be a PCOS subgroup.

Idiopathic hirsutism. A woman whose excessive hair growth has no known medical cause is said to have idiopathic hirsutism. Regularly menstruating women who have excess body hair characteristic of an ethnic group receive this diagnosis, as do regularly menstruating women with excess hair caused by increased sensitivity of the hair follicles to male hormone levels. Such women show no evidence of elevated testosterone levels, even on repeated testing, and their menstrual cycles are regular and frequently ovulatory. The incidence of idiopathic hirsutism in a large group of hirsute women has been put at 5 percent.

HAIRAN syndrome. Hyperandrogenism-insulin resistant-acanthosis nigricans (HAIRAN) syndrome results in symptoms of excess body hair, *marked* insulin resistance, and areas of skin pigmentation. About 3 percent of hirsute women have this syndrome. The changes occur early in puberty, typically with very high insulin levels and very dark acanthosis nigricans, particularly on the nape of the neck, under the arms, and in the groin area. This syndrome may be genetically associated with very severe insulin resistance, for which early diagnosis and treatment can be helpful.

High prolactin level (hyperprolactinemia). Women with hyperproclactinemia and PCOS are regarded by some physicians as a subgroup. The incidence of significant hyperprolactinemia in PCOS varies from 7 to 20 percent. The hormone prolactin, secreted by the pituitary gland, stimulates milk production after childbirth. It also stimulates progesterone production by the corpus luteum in the ovary. A high prolactin level results in overproduction of milk and can disrupt the menstrual cycle by blocking the action of FSH or LH. Some drugs can cause a high prolactin level, and your doctor will explore that as a possible cause. If the prolactin level is sufficiently high, an MRI of the head can exclude the presence of a small prolactin-secreting pituitary growth (adenoma). The drugs bromocriptine (Parlodel) and cabergoline (Dostinex) have been used successfully for hypersecretion states of prolactin. The effects of excessive production of prolactin may cause menstrual abnormalities, the absence of periods, acne, hirsutism, and occasional hair loss, all of which are readily treatable.

Cushing's syndrome. Any fairly rapid weight gain of more than twenty-five to thirty pounds in a year; high blood pressure; wide, violet-colored stretch marks; development of a significant fat pad on the back of the neck; round facial features; possible diabetes; acne; hirsutism; muscle weakness; and a lack of periods can be caused by excessive production of the stress hormone cortisol by the adrenal glands. This is called Cushing's syndrome. Extensive testing by an experienced endocrinologist is required for its diagnosis.

Testosterone-secreting neoplasm of ovaries or adrenal glands. A rapid weight change, markedly increased hirsutism or acne, thinning scalp hair, deepening of voice, a noticeable increase in muscle mass, and usually an absence of periods indicate a possible testosterone-secreting neoplasm (usually benign) of the ovaries or adrenal glands. The testosterone level is usually very high (greater than 150 mg/dL, and often greater than 200 mg/dL). A pelvic ultrasound is needed to check the ovaries for any sign of a growth. A CT scan of the adrenal glands using iodine contrast can help locate the neoplasm. Some doctors recommend an

MRI of the abdomen, but it's of little practical help in defining subtle changes in the ovaries that show up much better on ultrasound performed by an experienced radiologist.

Thyroid function abnormality. Thyroid function tests are used routinely in health assessments of women of reproductive age. They have limited usefulness, however, in helping to establish a diagnosis of PCOS. An *underactive* thyroid may cause heavy menstrual cycles and hair loss. On the other hand, an *overactive* thyroid is often associated with a decrease in menstrual flow, longer intervals between cycles, skin itchiness, hyperactivity, palpitations, and some hair loss.

Other conditions. Changes in weight and eating patterns can frequently cause hormonal changes. Drugs and moderate or severe stress can also affect hormones. Low levels of the ovary-stimulating pituitary hormones LH and FSH, usually with a low estrogen level, can indicate hypothalamic amenorrhea. This condition is characterized by reduced ovary stimulation by brain hormones and can have various causes, including poor eating habits and excessive exercise. On the other hand, high LH and FSH levels, with a low estrogen level, can be characteristic of women who have a relatively early onset of menopause, with symptoms such as hot flashes, insomnia, and lack of periods.

How an Endocrinologist Can Help You

Many women spend years suffering from their symptoms while searching for an adequate diagnosis and appropriate treatment. Early recognition of PCOS and immediate treatment by a specialist can save women much heartbreak and wasted effort. Diagnosis is difficult, however. It's no surprise that endocrinologists familiar with the condition are the most likely to recognize it at an early stage as well as the warning signs of insulin resistance and the insidious approach of type 2 diabetes.

Detection and treatment of blood lipid abnormalities are the first steps in avoiding cardiovascular disease. If you have unhealthy cholesterol or triglyceride levels, your specialist will probably suggest dietary measures and exercise. If they don't work, you may need a statin (for example, Lipitor), fibrate (Tricor), or niacin.

High blood pressure is called a silent killer because it often shows no symptoms, goes undetected, and can be dangerous. Your specialist can detect and treat it. Insulin resistance, blood lipid abnormalities, and high blood pressure can interact as a complex network of risk factors in the insulin resistance syndrome, to which women with PCOS are especially vulnerable.

When you know for certain that PCOS is responsible for your infertility, your specialist can almost certainly remedy the situation with highly successful medications, as discussed in chapter 10. Likewise, when your specialist knows that your skin or hair problems are caused by PCOS, he or she can prescribe medications for the symptoms that have been highly successful in clinical practice. We discuss these medications in chapter 11.

An experienced specialist will emphasize controlled eating patterns and exercise, offer you encouragement when you need it, and monitor your progress over the course of treatment. He or she will explain why lifestyle modification is essential to easing symptoms. You can make a good start with the PCOS diet program in the next chapter.

[6]

Right Foods, Right Way

As we've seen, nearly 75 percent of women with PCOS are overweight or obese, and frequently store that excess weight around their abdomens. Women who struggle with weight issues may feel they are weak, lack willpower, or have a psychological block that makes taking off just a few pounds seem like a task of epic proportions. This problem is especially common in women with PCOS, whose bodies often resist losing weight.

If the last paragraph describes you, take heart. A new approach combines the right foods with the right strategies—and it's been successful for women with PCOS. The purpose of this chapter is twofold: (1) to give you the right foods to help you lose weight and (2) to supply you with the right strategies to help keep the weight off without hunger or deprivation. In chapter 7 we get around to eating the real food.

This chapter will help you gain an appreciation of optimal eating for weight control, showing you how to keep many of your favorite foods. Perhaps most significantly, the benefits you can derive from this book's approach can last a lifetime. The eating plans and strategies will help you lose the weight you want and then will show you how to keep it off—all without feeling hungry or deprived. The latest research, some of which points to the role of genes in PCOS-related weight gain, can be overcome with a sound eating plan based on smart food strategies. It's important to remember that *genes impel; they don't compel*. With the right food management strategies, almost anyone suffering from PCOS can take control of her eating, her genetic influence, her metabolic resistance and, most importantly, her weight.

For what you will read in this chapter and the next, I am grateful for the direct participation of two health professionals whose knowledge in this area is much greater than my own. Stephen Gullo, Ph.D., contributed the concept of how foods affect us individually and why successful weight loss programs need to take into account the foods we have a history of abusing. President of the Institute for Health and Weight Sciences' Center for Healthful Living in New York City, he is the author of the book *The Thin Commandments* (Rodale, 2005). The glycemic index, meal plans, recipes, and much else were contributed by Martha McKittrick, R.D., C.D.N., C.D.E. A staff dietitian at The New York Presbyterian Hospital for the past twenty years, she also counsels individuals in her private practice, physicians, corporations, and health clubs, and appears on numerous television, radio, and webcast programs. In my medical practice, both coordinate with me in the nutritional care of women with PCOS, so I know firsthand what healing wonders their nutritional counseling can produce.

Since many women with PCOS have trouble losing weight when their diet contains high or sometimes even moderate amounts of carbohydrates—especially the high-glycemic variety— it's important that you follow a low-glycemic carbohydrate eating plan, eat small meals through out the day (three meals and two snacks are preferable), and always include some protein when you eat carbohydrates. Protein helps slow the absorption of sugar into the bloodstream. This program is ideal for women suffering from PCOS. It is based on low-fat protein; non-starchy green and white vegetables; fish oils from cold-water fish and seafood; white meat poultry; eggs and egg substitutes; low-fat, high-calcium dairy; cinnamon; and limited amounts of certain fruits.

We'll show you not only how to lose weight, but how to keep it off. You'll discover how to learn from your mistakes and not to feel defeated by them. Many women with PCOS who lose weight and gain it right back do so not because they're planning to fail, but because they're failing to plan. On the pages that follow you'll learn unique, creative strategies that have worked for thousands of women with long histories of yo-yo dieting—many PCOS sufferers who have long despaired about ever achieving control over their weight.

As you read more, you'll see how the strategies and eating plans reinforce one another. Your eating behavior and habits and the type of foods you choose are both critical for your long-term success at weight control. Whether you can change your genetic response to food is as yet unknown. However, your "metabolic resistance" to weight loss, as well as the sight, smell, taste, and texture of the foods that have sabotaged your weight, can be dramatically altered.

You simply need the right foods—the right way.

PCOS-FRIENDLY FOODS

Food is a critical player in the PCOS drama. All the foods we eat have a direct impact on our hormonal system, and since it's now known that the underlying cause of PCOS is an imbalance of sex hormones, the foods you eat can have an enormous impact on PCOS. The imbalance in PCOS patients is often linked with the way their bodies process insulin, the hormone that controls the amount of glucose that enters their cells. Many PCOS patients have too much insulin in their blood.

As you have read previously, many women with PCOS are insulin resistant, which makes it easy for them to put on weight that, unfortunately, is difficult to lose. Constantly fluctuating blood sugar levels often lead to food cravings, especially for carbohydrates, and elevated insulin levels cause the body to store more calories as fat. A recent study showed that women with PCOS are 40 percent less responsive to the hormones that help metabolize fat than healthy women, regardless of their weight.

For most people, thermogenesis (the rate at which food is metabolized) accounts for a large percentage of calorie burning after a meal. Thermogenesis is often greatly reduced in women with PCOS—their bodies simply do not burn up calories as quickly as those who do not have PCOS. As a result, their bodies store more of the calories from the foods they eat.

Another reason that the type of food you're choosing is so essential in managing PCOS is that your weight and your percentage of body fat are factors in determining the severity of your symptoms. So weight management may be one of the most powerful ways for you to reduce the negative impact of PCOS and its symptoms in your life.

Studies have shown that the PCOS symptoms respond remarkably well to dietary changes. Overweight women with PCOS who lose weight have a corresponding decline in testosterone levels and their symptoms decrease. The loss of 5 to 7 percent of total body weight can cause more than two-thirds of women to resume ovulating, even some with long histories of infertility.

WHAT KIND OF EATING PLAN
WORKS BEST FOR YOU?

Many women are "fat phobic" and will go to any length to avoid consuming fat. Their diets consist mainly of grains (often refined grains), veggies, fruits, and lean protein, as well as a plethora of fat-free products—salad dressings, cheeses, ice cream, cookies, and so on. Not uncommonly, these women have frequent cravings and fluctuating energy levels. Others are "carb phobic," with diets that contain large amounts of protein and fat but are almost devoid of carbohydrates, with the exception of low-carb products such as protein bars and other low-carb snacks. Many of these women report low energy levels.

Neither of these diets is ideal. Balanced meals work best in helping the majority of women control carb cravings, increase energy levels, and lose weight. By *balanced,* I mean meals that contain protein, fat, and carbs. Protein and fat help keep you feeling full longer. In addition, when eaten together with carbohydrates, they slow the rise and fall of blood sugar. The more gradual the rise in blood sugar, the less insulin your body produces. Carbohydrates provide your body with energy, so consuming too few carbs can cause headaches and low energy levels in some people. This is especially important if you exercise on a regular basis. Eating balanced meals can help keep your blood sugar stable for a longer period of time. This, in turn, can control hunger, decrease cravings, and promote better mood and energy levels.

The typical low-fat, high-carbohydrate weight loss diet is not the best choice for obese, insulin-resistant women. The majority of women with PCOS have more success in losing weight on a lower glycemic index diet. This is a diet plan that causes fewer sharp rises and falls of blood sugar.

Eating "healthier" carbs rather than sugary or refined carbs, as well as eating fewer carbohydrates overall, will reduce insulin secretion. Decreasing insulin levels can help to alleviate many of the symptoms of PCOS, including hunger and cravings. However, this does not mean that all women with PCOS need to be on a low-carb diet. Women who are lean and only slightly insulin resistant can do just as well on a nutritionally balanced diet that is moderate in carbs—again, focusing on "healthier" carbs. Bottom line: You need to find a plan that works best for you.

Some subjective indicators that the diet is working:

- decreased cravings
- increased energy levels

Some objective measures that the diet is working:

- weight loss
- decreased insulin levels
- more regular periods

There is no one-size-fits-all approach to the following plans. We all have different food likes and dislikes, and your lifestyle—whether you're a stay-at-home mom or a frequent business traveler who rarely eats a home-cooked meal—affects your eating habits. Some of us are more active than others, which affects our caloric needs as well as the nutrient composition of our diet. In addition, our bodies do not respond in the same way to the same foods. For example, some women can incorporate moderate-sized portions of carbohydrates such as pasta and bread into their diets without triggering cravings or the urge to eat more. Other women find that these same foods set off intense cravings or leave them feeling unsatisfied. Obviously, you want to avoid foods that cause uncontrollable cravings for more. Pay attention to how your body feels after eating and make adjustments to establish a plan that works for you.

SELECT LOWER GLYCEMIC INDEX CARBOHYDRATES

Carbohydrates in food break down into sugar in your blood. For example, when you eat pasta, the flour from the pasta breaks down into glucose. This provides you with energy. The same thing happens when you eat a piece of fruit, drink a glass of milk, or eat jelly beans. All are converted to blood sugar. Your body then releases insulin to control the level of sugar in your blood.

In the past, it was believed that simple carbohydrates (called sugars) caused a more rapid rise of blood sugar than complex carbohydrates (called starches). However, recent research shows that this is not always the case. Not all foods that are chemically similar (for example, starches) necessarily affect blood sugar levels in the same way. For example, white rice causes a higher blood sugar response than white pasta. Potatoes can cause an even higher blood sugar response—similar to the response after eating table sugar. The carbohydrates that release sugar quickly into the bloodstream are the ones that cause sudden surges in insulin. Over time, those high surges of insulin can cause the body to become insulin resistant. Eventually that insulin resistance can lead to diabetes and other related illnesses. Health experts now understand that all carbohydrates are not the same, and that our bodies do not treat them in the same manner.

Glycemic index. The glycemic index (GI) measures how quickly a particular carbohydrate affects blood sugar levels. The higher the number, the quicker the rise in blood sugar. In general, starchy foods like refined grain products (for example, white rice) and potatoes have a high glycemic index. Milk, many fruits, and non-starchy vegetables such as greens have a low glycemic index, while whole grains, peas, and other legumes have a moderate or low glycemic index.

Glycemic load. The glycemic load (GL) assesses the impact of carbohydrates on blood sugar. It gives a more comprehensive picture than the glycemic index because it takes into account how much available carbohydrate is in a serving of food. Available carbohydrates are those that provide energy (starch and sugar), but not fiber. Foods that have a low GL almost always have a low GI. For more information on the glycemic index and glycemic load, check out www.mendosa.com. This Web site also lists the glycemic index and glycemic load of various carbohydrate-containing foods.

BENEFITS OF A LOW GLYCEMIC INDEX DIET

The majority of insulin resistant people find it easier to lose weight on a lower glycemic index diet. They report feeling more satiated, with fewer cravings and better energy levels. This is likely due to the lower glycemic index foods causing a slower rise of blood sugar, followed by a slower drop, which produces less insulin than rapid fluctuations. As we have already discussed, high levels of insulin can contribute to cravings, hunger, and fat storage.

Low glycemic diets contribute to better health in other ways:

- The Nurses' Health Study found a relationship between high glycemic index diets and heart disease in women who were overweight or insulin resistant.
- Other studies suggest that high glycemic index foods may contribute to overeating and weight gain.
- Data from the Nurses' Health Study also suggested that women who ate the least amount of foods with a high glycemic intake had a 50 percent lower risk of diabetes than those who ate the most.
- A study conducted by the American Institute for Cancer Research found that the women who ate the least amounts

of high glycemic index carbohydrates were more than twice
as likely *not* to have breast cancer as those who ate the most.

Glycemic Index Limitations.

While the glycemic index can be a useful tool, keep in mind that
it does have some limitations.

In assigning a number to a food, the glycemic index as-
sumes that the food is eaten alone. In reality, however, we rarely
eat a single food by itself. You don't just have a baked potato for
dinner. When other foods are eaten at the same time, the
glycemic index of the particular food can change. Fat and fiber
slow the process of digestion and thus lower the glycemic index
of each of the foods involved. For example, a baked potato eaten
alone causes a rapid rise of blood sugar. However, the rise is not
as quick if you add a piece of broiled salmon and salad with olive
oil, because the potato is digested more slowly.

The glycemic index is affected by how the food is processed, the way it is prepared or stored, and its ripeness. For example, pasta cooked al dente (firm) is absorbed more slowly
than pasta that is overcooked. Another example: A banana that
is barely ripe has a lower glycemic index than a very ripe banana.

The glycemic index of a food is an average of how many
people respond to that food. Responses can be highly individual,
so it is important for you to pay attention to how you feel after
eating a particular food. For example, a sweet potato has a fairly
low glycemic index, but if you do not find sweet potatoes especially filling or you have cravings soon after eating them, it's best
to avoid them.

Keep good nutrition in mind when using the glycemic index. Just because peanut M&M's have a lower glycemic index
than carrots does not mean they are a good snack choice!

TIPS TO LOWER THE GLYCEMIC RESPONSE OF YOUR DIET

- Limit or avoid sugary foods and drinks, as well as refined or heavily processed carbohydrates such as sugary sodas and white bread.
- Consume all carbohydrates in moderation. Although eating carbs with a lower glycemic index is recommended, eating large portions of that carbohydrate can still trigger excessive insulin surges.
- Select whole grains (whole wheat pastas, brown rice, wild rice, whole rye) over refined grains (plain pasta, white bread).
- Select higher fiber foods. Compare food labels to find the higher fiber product. Select whole grain breads, pasta, and crackers with at least 3 grams of fiber, and cereals with at least 5 grams of fiber per serving. Government guidelines recommend 25 to 30 grams of fiber a day; the average person takes in only 11 grams!
- Try to eat four or five moderate-sized meals or snacks as opposed to two or three large meals.
- Adding a little fat to a meal can lower the glycemic response. Focus on heart-healthy fats such as olive and canola oils, avocado, nuts, and nut butters. But remember portion control, because all fats are high in calories!
- Craving mashed potatoes? Try mashed yams, mashed turnips, or cauliflower.

You may see different glycemic index ratings for the same food if you check one list against another. Here's why: There are two different glycemic index lists. One uses sugar as a benchmark, and the other uses white bread. The benchmark value of 100 is the standard against which all other foods on the index are measured. Experts could compile glycemic indexes based on orange juice (or honey, or some other food) as the benchmark of 100, and generate yet another set of values. The food scientists who created the existing indices chose sugar and white bread as benchmarks because they are two of the most widely consumed refined carbs. Both lists are valid and reliable for our purpose— just select the foods with a lower glycemic index number.

The following glycemic index uses white bread as a benchmark of 100. Also, as previously discussed, you may want to use the glycemic load, in place of the glycemic index, as a guide when selecting your carbohydrates.

Glycemic Index of Foods, Ranked from High to Low

A food with a glycemic index of less than 55 is considered a low glycemic food, while 56 to 69 is moderate and over 70 is considered high. Most non-starchy vegetables have a very low glycemic index.

Food	GI	Food	GI
Jelly beans	114	Sweet potato	54
Rice cakes	110	Pumpernickel bread	50
Dates	103	Oat bran	50
Baked potato	98	Bulgur	48
French baguette	95	Oat bran bread	48
Instant white rice	90	Mixed-grain bread	48
Pretzels	83	Carrots	47
Cornflakes	83	Orange	43
White bread	78	All-Bran cereal	42
Corn	78	Plums	39
Waffles	76	Apple	38
Graham crackers	74	Pasta	35 to 55
Kaiser roll	73	Skim milk	32
Watermelon	72	Peanut M&M's	32
Boiled potato	70	Soy milk	31
Pineapple	66	Protein-enriched spaghetti	28
Cantaloupe	65	Legumes	25 to 45
Raisins	64	Grapefruit	25
Wild rice	57	Barley, pearled	25
Banana	56	Cherries	22
Brown rice	55	Low-fat yogurt, artificially	
Slow-cooked oats	55	sweetened	14

WHAT ABOUT LOW-CARB PRODUCTS?

Take a walk down the aisles in your local supermarket and you will be surrounded by packaged foods proclaiming their low-carb status—breads, cereals, salad dressings, candy bars, and so forth. Terms such as *net carbs* and *impact carbs* can be confusing to someone trying to watch her carbohydrate intake. Are these products really better than the regular product? The answer is . . . sometimes.

In response to the rising popularity of low-carb diets, food manufacturers have come up with their own definitions of what constitutes low carb. Unfortunately, the FDA has not set up regulations for low-carb claims as it has done for low-fat and low-sodium claims. In calculating *net* or *impact* carbs, most manufacturers take the total amount of carbs a product contains and subtract the fiber and sugar alcohols, as well as other ingredients such as glycerine or glycerol. It is thought that these ingredients, which are carbohydrates, have less of an impact on blood sugar. While it is true that some sugar alcohols have less of an impact on blood sugar levels than other carbohydrates, it is untruthful to say that sugar alcohols as a group have no affect on blood sugar whatsoever.

Sugar alcohol or polyols are hydrogenated carbohydrates that are used in foods mainly as bulking agents (to give foods texture) or sweeteners. Examples include sorbitol, mannitol, maltitol, and xylitol. Sugar alcohols are incompletely absorbed from the small intestine and provide 0.2 to 3.0 kcal/gram compared with the usual 4 kcal/gram provided by other carbohydrates. At this time, the FDA requires that food manufacturers count sugar alcohols as 2 kcal/gram. In short, sugar alcohols are not calorie free. Their glycemic effect varies according to type and your unique response to them. They also can cause gas or have a laxative effect in some individuals.

Glycerol or glycerine is chemically characterized as a polyol (sugar alcohol) with 4 kcal/gram. It is used in a variety of products, including nutrition or energy bars and frozen desserts. At this time, the FDA requires the glycerin content to be included in the total carbohydrate content.

Do fewer carbs mean fewer calories? In some cases, low-carb products do have fewer carbs than the regular version. Manufacturers can lower the carbohydrate content of a product by:

- substituting soy and wheat protein for flour.
- adding fiber from wheat bran and oat bran.
- adding high-fat ingredients such as oil and nuts, and decreasing the amount of carbohydrates.
- replacing sugar with sugar alcohols and artificial sweeteners.

However, this does not mean that low-carb products are lower in calories. As a matter of fact, many of the lower carb products have just as many calories as the regular version. For example, a slice of "low-carb" Atkins bread has 60 calories and 8 grams of total carbs—although a claim is made for only 3 net impact carbs. In comparison, a slice of conventional "diet" bread typically has 50 calories and 10 grams of carbs. Not a significant difference.

Tips to help you through the low-carb maze. The fact that a product's label says it is low-carb does not necessarily mean that it is low-carb, low-calorie, or even healthful.

- **Note the serving size.** People often eat a whole bag thinking it is one serving, only to find out later it contained four servings!
- **Pay attention to the total caloric content.** Calories are still the most important factor when it comes to weight control. Even if a food is low in carbohydrates, it may not be low in calories, or a healthful choice.

- **When choosing between two products, select the one with the higher fiber content.** This is important when it comes to selecting cereals, breads, crackers, and so forth, because they can vary tremendously in fiber content. Higher fiber foods tend to have a lower glycemic index than lower fiber foods. In addition, fiber is important for good health.
- **Look for fat content, especially saturated fat content.** When the carb content is decreased, the fat content often increases. For example, compare the Skinny Cow Silhouette Fat Free Fudge Bar, which has 100 calories, 22 grams of carbs, and 0 grams of fat, to the Atkins Indulge frozen ice-cream bar, which contains 180 calories, 12 grams of carbs, and 16 grams of fat (12 of these fat grams are saturated). Some of you might select the Indulge bar because of its lower carb content. However, that would not be my recommendation in view of its high calorie and fat (especially saturated fat) contents.

If you're counting grams of carbs. Some of you following low-carb diets may be interested in counting grams of carbs. (Not everyone needs to do this!)

- **Fiber.** Since fiber has a minimal effect on raising blood sugar, some health care practitioners have suggested subtracting the grams of fiber from the total carbohydrate content if the product contains *5 grams of fiber or more*. This technique is often used by diabetics who take insulin. Many food manufacturers subtract the fiber content from the total carbohydrates even if the amount of fiber is as few as 1 to 2 grams. Don't make the same mistake!
- **Sugar alcohol.** If the product contains sugar alcohol, you can subtract half the grams of sugar alcohol from the total carbohydrate content.

- **Glycerol or glycerine.** If the product contains glycerol or glycerine, you need to include those grams in the total carbohydrate content.

DESIGNING YOUR MEAL PLANS

When planning your diet, keep good nutrition in mind rather than just focusing on calories, fats, or carbs. Think balance, variety, and moderation! A healthy diet is one that incorporates foods from the following groups:

Fruits and vegetables. Most fruits and vegetables are low in fat and are loaded with vitamins, minerals, fiber, and disease-fighting phytochemicals. Vegetables are low in calories and are a great way to fill yourself up. Aim for a minimum of 1½ cups of vegetables a day. Although fruit contains a moderate amount of calories and carbs, you can include 1 to 2 servings a day into your diet. See below for serving sizes and nutritional content of some fruits. We recommend that you select fruits with a lower glycemic index (or load).

Fruits: Each serving has approximately 60 calories and 15 grams of carbs.

1 small apple (4 oz)	½ cup unsweetened applesauce
¾ cup blueberries	½ cup canned fruit in its own juice
½ large grapefruit	⅓ small cantaloupe
1¼ cup strawberries	1 cup cubed melon
½ small mango	3 dates or 3 dried prunes
1 small or ½ large pear	1½ dried figs
12 grapes or 12 cherries	1 small nectarine
½ medium banana	¾ cup fresh pineapple
1 medium peach	4 whole, fresh apricots
2 small tangerines	1 small orange
2 small plums	

Starches and whole grains. Whole grains provide essential vitamins, minerals, antioxidants, fiber, and phytochemicals. The trouble is trying to figure out what *is* a whole grain and what's not. Look for a *whole* or *whole grain* before the grain's name in the ingredient list on the food label. For example, choose *whole grain wheat bread* over *white* or *"wheat" bread*. Products labeled as *multigrain, stoneground, seven-grain, pumpernickel*, or *organic* may actually contain little or no whole grains. Examples of whole grains include whole wheat, whole barley, whole oats, bulgur, quinoa, Kamut, spelt, buckwheat, wheat berries, and amaranth. You can also look for a "whole grain" claim on other parts of the package's label. For qualifying foods, the federal government has approved a health claim that recognizes the health benefits associated with diets rich in whole grains. This claim makes it easier for you to identify foods that are rich in whole grains. The health claim states:

> Diets rich in whole grain foods, and other plant foods and low in total fat, saturated fat, and cholesterol, may help reduce the risk of heart disease and certain cancers.

Even if you are following a low-carb diet, you can still fit several servings of whole grains into your diet. See below for serving sizes and nutritional content of starches.

Starches: Each serving has approximately 80 calories and 15 grams of carbs.

Low to moderate glycemic index choices—recommended:
The following breads should be *whole* or *whole grain.*

1 slice bread (1 ounce)
½ English muffin
2 slices diet bread
½ of a 6-inch pita
½ cup cooked oatmeal, slow-cooked
¾ cup whole grain cereal (about ¾ ounce)
½ cup of pasta (whole wheat)
½ cup pasta, protein enriched
⅓ cup wild brown rice
½ cup bulgur

½ cup barley

½ cup buckwheat

½ cup legumes (kidney beans, navy beans)

½ cup sweet potato

½ cup peas

Higher glycemic index choices—consume less frequently:
Any of the above bread choices that are not whole grain ("wheat," white, semolina).

¼ bagel (1 ounce)

1 mini (3-inch) pita

1 waffle, 4 inches across

½ small bagel (1 ounce)

½ cup mashed potato

1 small potato (3 ounces—looks like a baby red potato) or ½ small baked potato

½ cup corn, 1 ear of corn on the cob

½ hamburger or hot dog bun

1 corn or flour tortilla, 6 inches across

⅓ cup couscous

½ cup plantain

Although I do not forbid any foods, I recommend that you select whole grains or lower glycemic foods as often as possible.

Calcium-rich foods. Only one-half of Americans get the calcium they need. You need adequate calcium to strengthen your bones and decrease the risk of osteoporosis. Calcium can also help lower your blood pressure and may play a role in preventing colon cancer. In addition, new research suggests that low-fat dairy products play a role in burning fat. Aim for 1,000–1,500 mg of calcium a day. If you cannot meet your needs with food, take a calcium supplement. Calcium-fortified products vary, so make a habit of reading food labels for calcium content.

Here are some calcium-rich food sources:

8 ounces milk (1% or nonfat) = 300 mg

8 ounces yogurt (nonfat or low fat) = 350 to 400 mg

1 ounce cheese = 200 mg

Canned sardines, 3 ounces, with the bones = 375 mg
Canned salmon with the bones = 170 mg
Leafy greens, ½ cup = 100 to 150 mg

Protein. Protein is an important component of every cell in the body. Your body uses protein to build and repair tissues and to make enzymes, hormones, and other body chemicals. Eating adequate protein at meals and snacks can increase feelings of fullness and decrease hunger in between meals. Try to select lean rather than high-fat sources of animal protein.

- *Very Lean and Lean Protein Foods contain 30 to 55 calories per ounce and 0 to 3 grams of fat per ounce.*
  Skinless poultry
  All fish and shellfish
  Beef: USDA Select or Choice grades of beef trimmed of fat, such as round, sirloin, flank, tenderloin, and ground round
  Pork: fresh ham, boiled ham, Canadian bacon, tenderloin, center loin chop
  Lamb: roast, chop, leg
  Veal: lean chop, roast
  Cheese: cottage cheese, nonfat or 1%, ¼ cup; grated Parmesan cheese, 2 tablespoons; fat-free cheese or cheese with less than 3 grams of fat per ounce
- *Medium-Fat and High-Fat Proteins contain 75 to 100 calories per ounce and 5 to 8 grams of fat per ounce.*
  Beef: most beef products, including ground beef, meat loaf, corned beef, short ribs, and Prime grades of meat such as prime ribs
  Pork: top loin, chop, spareribs, ground pork, pork sausage
  Lamb: rib roast, ground
  Veal: cutlet (ground or cubed)
  Poultry: dark meat with skin, or fried chicken

Fish: fried fish

Cheese: regular cheeses such as American, Swiss, and cheddar have 100 calories per ounce; cheeses such as feta and part-skim mozzarella have 70 calories per ounce

Others: eggs, sausage, salami, hot dogs, bacon, knockwurst

Nut butters: 1 tablespoon

Tofu, 4 ounces or ½ cup

Despite being higher in calories and total fat than some other protein foods, nut butters and tofu contain more unsaturated than saturated fat. They also have many health benefits.

Fats. Not all fats are created equal! The type of fat you consume is more important than the amount of fat. Certain types of fat can damage your health, whereas others offer health benefits. Keep in mind that while some fats are more healthful than others, they all have about the same amount of calories. Your fat cells do not know the difference between "good" or "bad"! Therefore, it is best to consume all fats in moderation to help control your caloric intake.

Limit These fats:

- *Saturated fats* are found in foods that come from animals, including whole milk and products made from whole milk (ice cream, cheese, butter, sour cream, etc.), chicken skin, and high-fat cuts of red meat. Some plant-derived foods, such as coconut and palm oil, also contain saturated fat. All these saturated fats can raise LDL ("bad") cholesterol. Since women with PCOS frequently have an abnormally high fat content in their blood, it makes sense to limit your intake of these fats.

- *Trans or hydrogenated fats:* Hydrogenated fats are found in stick margarine and shortening, some soft tub margarines, many processed foods, snack foods (including potato chips), cookies, crackers, commercial baked desserts, and fried fast foods. Hydrogenated fats contain trans fatty acids (TFAs) that act much like saturated fats in that they can raise LDL cholesterol. In addition, they can decrease HDL ("good") cholesterol. Manufacturers don't advertise the presence of these fats, so check the ingredient list for the words *hydrogenated fat* and avoid products containing trans fats as much as possible

Select Healthy Fats:
- *Monounsaturated fats* are found in olive oil, rapeseed oil, many nuts and nut butters, and avocados. These fats, when substituted for saturated fats and TFAs, can help to decrease your risk of heart disease. I recommend nuts and nut butters as part of meals and snacks—assuming you can control the portions!
- *Omega-3 fats* are found in fatty fish, including salmon, tuna, mackerel, trout, and sardines, as well as in flaxseeds, canola oil, and walnuts. Omega-3 fats have anti-clotting properties and anticlotting effects, which protect the heart and may suppress tumor growth. Try to include fatty fish (as well as all kinds of fish!) in your diet at least three times a week.

WINNING STRATEGIES

As well as eating PCOS-friendly foods, your long-term healthful lifestyle plans should take into account what works best for you, physically and emotionally. What has worked best for you in the past is likely to do so in the future. The same is true for trouble spots. What caused problems for you in the past is likely to trip you up again! You have a history that you need to consider in order to make a plan that's going to work.

Learn to Think Historically, Not Just Calorically

Every medical student learns that the first step in assessing a new patient's health is taking a personal history. Yet when it comes to dieting and weight control, personal history is often entirely ignored. This problem has unknowingly led millions of dieters to failure, as the same people gain back the same weight with the same foods again and again.

Anyone who has ever tried losing weight has been taught that they need to burn more calories than they take in. Or that they need to count the grams of fat or carbohydrates in the foods they eat. Yet it's this emphasis on calorie and carbohydrate counting alone that has led millions of dieters to failure. The single most powerful strategy of winners at weight control is taking their food history into account.

Thinking calorically (about the calories alone) puts the focus squarely on food and how it functions in the body. Thinking *historically* shifts the focus to you—how you have behaved toward food, and your unique history (or eating print) with a food or group of foods. When you stop thinking calorically and start thinking historically, you shift your focus to the most critical element for success at weight control: *you.*

Two people may react very differently to the same food. For one person, a single dinner roll may be very satisfying, especially if that person has no history of abusing bread. Another person might only have to take a bite of that very same roll for it to unleash a torrent of cravings that will cause her to consume the entire bread basket. Or she might find herself thinking more and more about bread, which could lead to ever greater quantities consumed at subsequent meals. Knowing which is true for you could mean the success or failure of your weight loss plan. Ultimately, it doesn't matter whether a roll has 200 or 300 calories. When you take a hard look at your history with a food, not just how many calories it contains, you change your thinking about it. Do you have a long history of abusing bread and bread products? Does even a taste lead to you eating thousands of calories' worth a short time later?

Thinking historically, not just calorically, is the first and most critical strategy for success at weight loss and, more importantly, long-term weight control. Once you start thinking about a food or group of foods in terms of your individual history with that food, your perception changes. You'll look at that harmless little roll and it will take on a whole new light. Try to think of the foods you have a negative history with in terms of *calorie units*. That is to say, instead of asking "How many calories?" ask yourself "How many of those do I typically eat at a sitting, based on my history?"

So, you see, when it comes to food, history always trumps calories. When people fail in dieting, it often has nothing to do with the particular plan, or their motivation. They fail because they include foods in their diet that they have a long history of abusing. Much has been made in the popular media of the benefits of eating whole grain products. That's fine if you have no history of abusing grain products. However, if your history says otherwise, then you're just setting yourself up for trouble.

How to Make Food History Work for You

It's been said that predictability is the highest goal of science, and I'm going to argue that knowing your own unique history with food is the most scientific approach to weight loss. Your food history does the following:

- It predicts in advance how you'll behave with any food.
- It predicts the time of day when you're most vulnerable and likely to lose control or overeat.
- It helps you evaluate food not just in terms of caloric intake and caloric release, but in terms of how it affects your behavior, mood, appetite and, ultimately, your success at dieting.

- It predicts the situations that you most often associate with out-of-control eating.
- It establishes guidelines and helps you set boundaries that don't come from some "one size fits all" approach to dieting, but from your own eating prints.
- It changes your thinking from "I'm good or I'm bad" to "What does or doesn't work for me?" Don't think about the foods the foods you can or can't have—think about the food that does or doesn't work for you.

Food Journaling

Your eating habits play a major role in how you feel physically and mentally—and, of course, whether you are losing weight. Although your total caloric intake is the most important factor when it comes to weight control, there are other factors that are important as well. The times you eat, the composition of your meals, and the kind of carbohydrates you are eating all play a role in your weight, mood, energy levels, and health. Before you start to work on your eating plan, it's important that you get a really good idea of what your eating habits are like and establish which areas you need to work on. I'm going to guess that right about now you're saying to yourself that you already know where your problem areas are. That you know how many calories you eat in a day. But have you kept a food journal? Have you weighed or measured your portions? Studies have shown that most people vastly underestimate the amount of food they eat. It is time to get out the measuring cups, spoons, and food scale.

Make a commitment to keep a food record for at least a week. Try the food diary format below. Feel free to make changes, and keep your diary in a notebook or online, whichever is easiest for you.

			SAMPLE FOOD DIARY			
Day:						
Time	Food or Beverage	Portion Size	Where	Mood/ Emotion	Degree of Hunger	Calories (and grams of carbs if desired)

As you can see, there's space to enter information about the following points.

- Time of day you eat
- What you eat, including portion size. Use a measuring cup for grains such as cereal, rice, and pasta (cooked), and a measuring spoon for oil, salad dressing, and peanut butter. Use a food scale for meat, fish, poultry, cheese, nuts, and dry pasta.

- Where you are when you eat. Certain places can trigger eating.
- Any emotion you feel before or while you're eating. Eating in response to emotions is a major cause of overeating for many of us.
- Degree of hunger. Before you eat, rate how hungry you are on a scale of 0 to 10, where 10 is famished and 0 is not hungry at all. A 5 is neutral: neither hungry nor not hungry.
- Record calories, if you wish.

Once you have kept your food record for a week or so, ask yourself these questions.

TIMING QUESTIONS
What times of the day do you normally eat?
Do you let more than four hours go between meals or snacks?
Do you generally plan a snack for the middle of the afternoon?
Do you skip meals?

PORTION CONTROL QUESTIONS
Did any of your portions surprise you?
Which foods do you tend to overeat?

COMPOSITION OF MEALS QUESTIONS
Are you including an adequate source of protein and fat at meals? (For example, do you try to make a meal of a salad with just veggies and fat-free dressing?)
Are you selecting whole grains or refined grains? (For example, whole wheat bread or white bread? Brown rice or white rice?)
Are you eating at least three servings of vegetables a day? One or two fruits? Two servings of dairy products?
Do certain foods cause increased cravings? If so, which foods?
Do you experience fatigue or increased cravings after eating high-carbohydrate meals?
Which snacks are most satisfying and help control your hunger?
Which snacks leave you wanting more?

Which kinds of meals or snacks make you feel better: higher protein or higher carb? For example, a high-carb meal like cereal, milk, and fruit or a high-protein omelet? Pretzels (high carb) or small handful of nuts (high protein)?

Think about what these questions reveal to you. Do you go for long stretches of time without eating? Do certain foods make you feel better than others? Do certain foods trigger you to eat more? Do you find that certain emotions frequently drive you to eat? Keep these thoughts in mind as you read on.

Reality Check

Studies have shown that women are now eating 335 more calories per day than they did in 1971, increasing their total caloric intake from 1,540 to 1,875 calories a day, with 40 percent of those calories eaten outside the home. That percentage seems low to me. Most of us have hectic schedules and tend to grab food on the run—a bagel or a muffin for breakfast, a deli sandwich for lunch, perhaps an afternoon snack from the vending machine. If you don't have time to cook dinner, it could be take-out pizza, Chinese food, or a "home-cooked" frozen meal. If you are following a low-carb diet, you may well be consuming too many calories from protein and fat, or maybe, like so many others, you've simply gotten into the habit of eating more calorie-laden foods of all kinds. Bottom line: All calories count, wherever you happen to eat them.

Calculate Your Caloric Needs

Whether you plan on counting calories, it is still a good idea to have an estimate of what your body needs to maintain your present weight and perhaps more importantly the changes you'll need to make to lose weight. Your caloric needs will vary depending upon several factors, including activity level, age, sex, weight, body composition, and individual metabolism. Many online caloric need calculators are available, such as at www.calorie control.org/calcalcs.html or www.active.com. Keep in mind that many online caloric calculators overestimate the caloric needs of obese women.

Here is a quick method for estimating your caloric needs.

FOR WEIGHT MAINTENANCE
10 calories per pound for women who are obese, very inactive, or chronic dieters

13 calories per pound for women over age fifty-five who are very active or moderately active women under the age of fifty-five

15 calories per pound for very active women under the age of fifty-five

If you tend to have a difficult time losing weight and are obese, very inactive, or a chronic dieter, it is possible that you may need to reduce your intake to 8 or 9 calories per pound.

FOR WEIGHT LOSS
To lose 1 pound a week, subtract 500 calories from maintenance caloric level

To lose 2 pounds a week, subtract 1,000 calories from maintenance calorie level

Thirty years old, 5 foot 5, and 160 pounds, Sue exercised three times a week for forty-five minutes. She had been "dieting" for many years, but the gains pretty much cancelled out the losses. To find her caloric needs for weight maintenance, Sue multiplied her weight by 12 (since was moderately active, yet a chronic dieter). Her weight maintenance caloric needs were approximately 1,920 calories a day. To lose a pound a week (subtract 500 calories), she needed to consume 1,420 calories a day. To lose one and a half pounds a week (subtract 750 calories), she needed to consume 1,170 calories.

Keep in mind that these are just calculations and they do not take your individual metabolism into account. Many overweight, insulin-resistant women with PCOS do not lose weight according to the preceding calculations. If you have been unable to lose weight on a low-fat or moderately low-carb, calorie-controlled diet, try the accelerated weight loss eating plans in this program. They average 1,100 calories a day, with approximately 35 percent of the calories coming from carbs.

ALL CALORIES COUNT!

To lose weight, you need to consume fewer calories than you burn. Many of the popular diet plans focus on restricting fat or carbs—perhaps to distract you from the fact that they're also reduced-calorie diets! As discussed, your body needs a certain amount of calories in order to maintain your current weight. If you eat fewer calories, you lose weight. If you can't limit your calories to a point below maintenance, you won't. It does not matter where the calories come from—excessive calories from protein, fat, or carbs will all stymie your weight loss goals.

Betty, who had PCOS, was insulin resistant and a chronic dieter. She had been following a very low carb diet for twelve weeks, had lost four pounds initially, but had been unable to lose any more weight. In fact, she gained two pounds back. She had frequent headaches and minimal energy, and soon she was making only two trips to the gym per week instead of her usual four.

Betty's breakfast consisted of two eggs, her midmorning snack was 2 ounces of cheese, and her lunch from a diner was a large burger (7 ounces, no roll). For an afternoon snack she grabbed a protein bar or a large, low-carb cookie and often ate a few ounces of cold cuts while making dinner—8 ounces of chicken, or fish and a cup of veggies with a tablespoon of oil. A few handfuls (2 ounces) of nuts made up her after-dinner snack. Betty's diet totaled approximately 2,200 calories. At a weight of 160 pounds with moderate activity, Betty only needed about 1,900 calories to maintain her weight and 1,400 calories to promote a one pound loss a week. The numbers, obviously, weren't working in her favor! While she'd successfully cut back on carbs, she'd unwittingly put herself on a diet guaranteed to result in a slow but steady weight gain! She was consuming an excessive amount of calories in the form of protein and fat. Too few carbs in her diet led to headaches, low energy levels, and fewer trips to the gym.

To help Betty lose weight, we cut her calories to a more balanced 1,400 a day. We cut down on her portion sizes of protein and fat, and added in some low glycemic index carbs in the form of fruit and whole grains. The changes were as follows:

> *Breakfast:* 3 egg whites made with ½ cup veggies sautéed in 1 teaspoon fat, and 1 slice of whole wheat toast
>
> *Midmorning:* 1 string cheese and a handful of baby carrots
>
> *Lunch:* grilled chicken kebab, 5 ounces, with a side of steamed veggies, 1 teaspoon fat
>
> *Afternoon snack:* 12 almonds and 1 small apple
>
> *Dinner:* 5 oz of lean protein, 1 tablespoon oil, 1½ cups veggies, and ½ cup brown rice
>
> *Snack after dinner:* 1 cup of berries with 2 tablespoons sugar-free whipped cream

Betty reported that her energy levels improved and her headaches disappeared. She went back to exercising four days a week and lost four pounds over the next month.

Low-Carb Diets and Water Loss

Some of you may be wondering why Betty initially lost four pounds and then regained two. Her initial weight loss on the scale was due to a loss of water. It is not unusual to lose several pounds in the first week of low-carb dieting. Here's how it works: Your body stores carbs in the form of glycogen to use for energy. Glycogen is stored in association with water. When you decrease your intake of carbs, your body uses the stored glycogen for energy. As the stored carbs are being burned, your body releases the water stored with it. This is why you probably find yourself running to the bathroom frequently when first starting a low-carb diet! It is not unusual to lose three pounds or more of water in the first week of following a low-carb diet, but ultimately, it's calories that count. To lose one pound of fat, you must create a deficit of 3,500 calories. In Betty's case, she did not have a caloric deficit. On the contrary, she was consuming more calories than her body needed. After her initial water weight loss, I would not have expected her to lose weight. Fortunately, the fix was a simple one: By cutting her caloric intake down to 1,400 while maintaining a

DO YOU KNOW HOW MANY CALORIES YOU CONSUME A DAY?

Here are some tips to help you become aware of your caloric intake.

On occasion, weigh and measure some foods. Do you know what one cup of pasta looks like? You would probably be surprised at how small it is. Do you know that an average restaurant-sized serving of pasta is 3 to 4 cups? That is 600 calories—before the sauce is added! Do you know that an average-size bagel (4 to 5 ounces) is equivalent to eating four to five slices of bread and has 360 calories?

The next time you slice off a piece of cheese for a snack, put it on your food scale first. Full-fat cheese is approximately 100 calories an ounce, whereas low-fat cheese ranges from 50 to 70 calories an ounce. And who eats just an ounce?

Measure or weigh your cold cereal. Most of us eat a larger serving size than what is listed on the label. It is not uncommon to eat a 300-calorie bowl of cereal (and that does not include the milk and fruit on top).

Is steak and a salad your idea of a "dieter's delight" in a restaurant? Think again—a 12-ounce Prime cut of steak can easily have 1,200 calories and 96 grams of fat, while the salad with blue cheese dressing (2 tablespoons) has 190 calories and 18 grams of fat. This is a grand total of 1,390 calories and 114 grams of fat!

Many chain restaurants list the nutritional content of their menu selections on their Web sites. Check to see if the restaurants you frequent have Web sites.

low glycemic index diet, she was able to lose about a pound a week. This was mainly from loss of body fat—not a water loss.

Be Calorie Smart

You do not have to feel deprived when trying to lose weight. These calorie-smart options can help fill you up while keeping your caloric intake on the low side:

- 6 ounces cooked shrimp (12 large) have 168 calories. Delicious and filling!
- 6 ounces cooked scallops have 175 calories. Try broiling them with lemon or cooking them in a nonstick pan with mushrooms and wine.
- 6 ounces skinless turkey breast has 180 calories.
- An egg white omelet made with 4 egg whites and 1 cup of veggies in a nonstick skillet only has 110 calories. Add flavor with a little hot sauce or salsa.
- Homemade vegetable soup made with low-fat chicken broth (low-sodium, if desired) and your favorite low-starch vegetables is a low-cal winner; 2 cups are only 50 calories or so. Read the labels for the nutrition content of commercial soups. Studies have shown that soup eaten before or as part of a meal can help to promote weight loss. Soup helps fill you up, as well as slow down the rate of eating.
- Vegetables—raw or cooked—are low-calorie winners. For variety, try them grilled, roasted, or stir-fried (see next chapter for recipes); 1½ cups of vegetables are 100 calories or less.

Caloric Content of Some Popular Foods

1 slice of pizza: 450 calories
Deli tuna salad sandwich: up to 730 calories
Caesar salad: 400 to 600 calories (more for entrée size)
General Tso's or kung pao chicken: over 1,500 calories and 60 grams of fat

MOOD EATING AND PCOS

Mood eating is about *immediately* replacing an unpleasant feeling with a pleasurable one. Much research has been done on the relationship between food and mood—for instance, on the connection between eating carbs and brain levels of the mood-enhancing neurotransmitter serotonin. Carbs may be responsible for the spike, but unfortunately the effects last for less than thirty seconds, and you then need to eat more carbs!

Mood eating is a vexing problem for dieters. It's also one of the more challenging issues to deal with because so many of the "one size fits all" diets on the market today have a few or no answers for people with a history of this condition. Diets that follow the calories-in–calories-out approach to weight loss often lose sight of the person—the key factor in any weight loss equation. In addition, mood eating is often intensified in women with PCOS because the emotional stress brought on by physical and metabolic changes often stirs up feelings of anxiety, fear, and frustration. Along with changes in their physical appearance and metabolism, women with PCOS are at increased risk for reproductive problems, including infertility, miscarriage, and diseases such as type 2 diabetes, heart disease, and uterine cancer. So it's no surprise that, taken together, these physical and emotional stresses can intensify the symptoms of PCOS.

If you have PCOS, you may find mood eating is most often triggered by day-to-day annoyances such as an argument with your spouse or getting stuck in traffic. These problems may simply seem magnified because of your condition. It's important to recognize that the type of stress that causes a person to mood eat is predictable—it often arises from the same situations such as interactions with an irritating coworker.

For most of us, mood eating is not about food in and of itself. It's almost always about snacking or grabbing on whatever food happens to be within arm's reach, particularly snack foods and simple carbohydrates such as pretzels, potato chips, and chocolate. For a lesser number, it's about a different type of snack food, such as ice cream.

What characterizes eating as mood eating?

- **Same food.** Are you returning again and again to your favorite snack foods? Mood eaters rarely react to stress or disappointment by food shopping or cooking a gourmet meal. Mood is about snacking on what's easiest to get in your mouth.
- **Same place.** Are you eating alone in your kitchen? Most mood eating takes place in the kitchen. A small number of mood eaters do their eating at work. The availability of snack foods in your home creates cravings, and the variety stimulates consumption.
- **Same time of day.** Are you snacking in the late afternoon or evening? Mood eating usually takes place at these times, and rarely occurs in the morning.
- **Same moods.** Are you eating because you feel anxious, bored, angry, betrayed, or frustrated? These feelings, which are common in women with PCOS, often trigger mood eating.
- **Same people.** Are certain people triggering your mood eating? The same people stress out mood eaters again and again. For PCOS patients, it could even be people who are trying to be supportive of your condition, such as a doctor, parent, spouse, or friend.
- **Same situations.** Are you snacking in response to certain situations? Mood eaters snack because the same situations stress them out again and again. Perhaps you reach for a snack before you visit the doctor, or, if you're trying to conceive, before you take a pregnancy test.
- **Same quantities of food.** Are you choosing snacks that enable you to drag out the eating experience, such as pretzels or a bag of M&M's? Mood eaters want the eating—the source of comfort—to last as long as possible.

- **Same reason.** Are the foods you're choosing providing you with a sense of comfort, or do you view them as a reward or treat? If you're distressed over your condition, you may turn to a favorite snack to allay your feelings, or decide to "treat" yourself if you've had a particularly difficult or stressful week.

The most immediate reason a person uses a food to change her mood is because it tastes really good. Mood eaters usually choose foods with a creamy or crunchy texture that's either sweet or salty. These tastes and textures provide the person with immediate gratification, in much the same way that exercising vigorously or talking with a friend about a personal problem can release pent-up feelings or emotions. If you keep a lot of snack foods around your house, eating to vent your emotions becomes markedly easier.

There's no denying that the foods most mood eaters choose have a pleasing taste. However, the pleasure derived from food is fleeting, and most mood eaters end up regretting it later. On the bright side, since mood eating is a learned behavior, it can just as easily be unlearned and corrected through strategy.

Strategies That Put an End to Mood Eating

Contrary to what you might think, the best place to end mood eating is *not* your therapist's office. It's the supermarket! Since mood eating often occurs in the kitchen and with foods you bring into the house, don't buy the snacks you tend to abuse when you're anxious or stressed. Even the most hardened mood eater will resort to another activity, such as reading or watching TV, if the snacks are not immediately accessible. Think about it. Are you really going to break the habit of snacking on potato chips or pretzels if there's a supply in your kitchen pantry?

Snacks that won't make you fat include cut-up green vegetables, apples, individually wrapped low-fat cheeses, chilled beverages such as flavored water or diet lemonade, sugar-free gum, single-serving bags of unsalted sunflower seeds, and bran crackers (especially GG Scandinavian Crisp bread crackers, which are great for killing appetite). You may also want to keep some low-calorie substitutes for your favorite foods on hand, such as an individually wrapped bag of Knight's lite popcorn, a Weight Watchers chocolate mousse pop, or a Van's 7-Grain Belgian Waffle.

Sometimes the availability of a favorite snack food creates a rationalization to eat it. The single best strategy to end mood eating is to throw out all the mood snacks in your home. The next time you go shopping, make a list and keep your mood snacks off it. If you live with someone and must keep snack foods around, especially those that tempt you or trigger cravings, buy only those snacks that come in single servings and hand them over to the person who wanted them as you're unloading the groceries.

- Keep an ample supply of snacks available that won't make you fat. If you're craving chocolate, you may find that one chocolate mousse pop leaves you satisfied. Remember to consider your history before you make a decision. If you feel that the waffle may stimulate cravings for baked goods, this may not be the best choice for you.
- Keep all snack foods out of sight.
- Ask family members not to snack in front of you.
- Have someone hide tempting snacks.
- If nothing else works, lock the most enticing snacks, except for the ones that are perishable, in a cash box. It may sound a little draconian, but it works. Remember: Availability creates cravings.
- Make a list of healthy, low-calorie snacks and shop for them. Banish things you have a history of problems with.
- Recognize trouble before it happens. If you have a weakness for french fries, don't drive by a McDonald's on a day when you expect to be under stress.

- Rehearse a stressful situation or event you expect to encounter. Many mood eaters find it helpful to mentally prepare for a stressful situation. For instance, you can practice what you're going to say to someone you're anxious about confronting, or visualize yourself breezing through a situation you dread, such as a visit to the doctor's office.
- Block that mood. The winners at weight control don't let the unknown catch them off-guard. *Planning is stronger than willpower*—this is a motto that all former mood eaters live by. Stress doesn't have to convert to body fat. One of the best strategies to end mood eating is talking on the telephone. *It's the quickest and most effective way to end mood eating immediately.* So call someone you enjoy talking to, such as a friend or colleague. You don't even have to tell the person why you're calling. Talking on the phone diverts your mind and will help relax you. It's a great blocking behavior. You may even find that by the time you finish your conversation, the compulsive need to overeat has passed.

There's much confusion about the difference between pleasure and happiness. Any pleasurable feeling you derive from food is transient. In fact, the pleasure you derive from a cookie or a bag of potato chips may actually destroy the possibility of lasting happiness. Even if you're feeling anxious or stressed, or are depressed about having PCOS, you're going to feel much better about yourself if you consistently make decisions about eating that will help you take control of your weight.

Any pain in your life that has resulted from PCOS will only be aggravated if the foods you have turned to for comfort have done little except cause you to gain weight. If you reach for food every time you to feel frustrated or angry over having PCOS, you'll be even more upset the next time you step on the scale or look in the mirror. *The great irony of mood eating is that we eat because something has upset or frustrated us and then we get even angrier after we abuse food because of it.*

Every time you use food as a crutch or eat in response to a stressful event, person, or situation, you perpetuate in your own psyche the very real sense of being unable to cope without food. It doesn't have to be that way. PCOS is not a life sentence. Adopting the strategies in this chapter and the eating plan in the next can help you from turning to food the next time you feel out of control or despondent about your condition. Having a plan puts you in the driver's seat, and there's no greater feeling in the world.

[7]

LET'S EAT

In this chapter I'll share Martha McKittrick's eating plan and recipes that my patients have followed with tremendous success. They will enable you to lose weight without having to abandon all of the foods you love. With this plan, success is not about deprivation, but substitution.

No matter what life throws at you, it will always be easier to handle if you're in control of your weight. Failing again and again to meet your weight loss goals, or feeling out of control in your life, can be totally reversed by everyday smart thinking, such as saying no to a bread basket, piece of cake, or bag of pretzels. To change your weight, you need to change your thinking. Let's get started.

FOUR STEPS TO EATING RIGHT

Here are some pointers to eating right, arranged in four steps. You need to pay attention to directions and amounts, and also to your body's reaction to what and how much you eat. If you have doctor's orders to avoid something, those orders override suggestions here. But it's not all about avoiding and saying no. Look for foods you like in the food lists provided in this chapter and enjoy them.

STEP 1: EMBRACE GOOD PRACTICES

Portion sizes are important. Unlike many popular low-glycemic diet plans, we focus on portion control and do not allow eating unlimited amounts of protein and fat. Therefore, you will need to weigh certain foods on a food scale and measure other foods in a measuring cup until you feel you can eyeball portions accurately.

- Use a food scale to weight cooked protein and cheese as well as dry pasta and potatoes, if you choose to incorporate these foods into your eating plan.
- Use a measuring cup to measure cooked starches, such as rice, oatmeal, and other grains.
- Use measuring spoons for oils and salad dressings.

Try not to skip meals and snacks. Eating small meals regularly helps control overeating.

Avoid alcohol. Not only is alcohol an empty source of calories, but it can also reduce your willpower to watch what you eat. In addition, it is not recommended that you drink alcohol if you are taking metformin (Glucophage). Therefore, alcohol should be saved for special occasions—and the metformin should not taken at the same time. Ideally, you should also account for the calories in alcohol by omitting calories from your eating plan. An average drink (6 ounces wine, 1½ ounces hard liquor) has about 100 calories. Avoid alcoholic beverages with sweet mixers, such as rum and Coke.

Take a multivitamin supplement. It is almost impossible to eat a perfectly nutritionally balanced diet, especially if you are on a reduced calorie diet. While real food is always best, a multivitamin can help provide your body with some of the nutrients your diet may be lacking. For women taking metformin, it is especially important to take multivitamins, because metformin can deplete or interfere with the absorption of vitamin B-12 and folic acid. Lastly, if you are not consuming 1,200 mg of calcium a day from food, I recommend that you take a calcium supplement.

Step 2: Make This about You

Pay attention to how your body feels after eating various foods. If you find a particular meal suggestion (for example, a breakfast of yogurt, bran cereal, and nuts) does not satiate you, omit that meal or snack from your eating plan and focus on the meals that do satisfy you (perhaps the egg white omelet with veggie sausage and light toast).

Customize. For more flexibility, we have included lists of approved starches grains, fruit, and nuts that you can substitute for foods listed in the meal plans. For example, if you do not like the fruit on the menu for Monday, feel free to choose another from the fruit list. The same goes for starches/grains and nuts. (Do not eat grapefruit if you are taking Lipitor or other statins.)

Don't forget your food history. If you have always had difficulty controlling portions of a certain food, for example, nuts or bread, do not include that food in your meal plan.

Eat your favorite foods. Many of my patients ask if they can incorporate some of their favorite "non-diet" foods into their eating plans on occasion. The answer is absolutely! No one should
feel deprived 100 percent of the time. Maybe plan to have a
moderate portion of your mother-in-law's famous lasagna at a
family get-together, or split a piece of cheesecake with your husband at your favorite restaurant. The key is that these indulgences need to be moderate, planned, and done only on special
occasions—I might suggest twice a month. However, if you are
trying our accelerated weight-loss plans, try to adhere to them
strictly for at least three weeks before adding treats. Lastly, if you
find that straying from the diet plans "sets you off," avoid
indulgences—or at least stick to those treats that do not trigger
uncontrolled eating.

Take your special needs into account. For those of you who
are trying to limit your sodium intake, make sure to read food labels. Some of the soups and cheese products in the My Favorite
Food section may contain fairly high amounts of sodium. Select
lower sodium products when available.

Step 3: Things to Enjoy

Use a cooking spray, instead of oil or butter, whenever you can.

Pile on the greens. Salad greens can be consumed in unlimited
amounts.

Most vegetables welcome. The following vegetables are low in
calories (approximately 50 calories per cup cooked) and fairly
low in carbs (approximately 6 to 8 grams per cup cooked):

artichoke hearts	bean sprouts
asparagus	broccoli
green beans	brussels sprouts

cabbage	pea pods
cauliflower	spinach
celery	summer squash
cucumber	tomatoes
eggplant	water chestnuts
green onions	zucchini
mushrooms	

While it is unlikely that anyone ever gained weight from eating too many green beans, on our accelerated weight loss program, we still recommend that you account for your calories from vegetables.

Drink plenty of fluids. Water, seltzer, diet drinks, regular and decaf tea, and regular and decaf coffee are all allowed. What you drink can have an effect on your health. It has been suggested that tea can help decrease the risk of cancer and heart disease. In addition, it may play a role in weight loss. For those of you who enjoy a cup of coffee, recent research has shown some health benefits as well. However, other studies have linked caffeinated beverages to increased insulin resistance. I, therefore, urge moderation in consumption of all caffeinated beverages, including coffee, tea, and diet sodas.

STEP 4: TROUBLESHOOTING

Hidden calories. Be careful with salad dressings. There is no easier way to ruin a healthful low-calorie meal than to top it with 300 calories of a dressing! Consume a maximum of 70 calories for salad dressing. Your choices include:

- 1½ teaspoons of oil and unlimited vinegar amounts to 70 calories.
- 2 tablespoons of light commercial dressing can range from 10 to 80 calories. Check the label, since calories vary widely.

- 1 tablespoon creamy commercial dressing can be 60 calories or more. Again, check the label. In a restaurant, if a light dressing is not available, order the regular dressing on the side and use only 1 tablespoon. Add extra vinegar if needed. You can do the same with your favorite higher calorie salad dressings at home.
- Your best bet is making your own dressing. You can keep the calories down by adding in more of the lower calorie ingredients (vinegar or buttermilk) and less oil of the higher calorie ingredients (oil or cheese).

FEEDING YOUR SWEET TOOTH

Artificial sweeteners are allowed—but moderation is best! Many women prefer the taste of Splenda. Word of caution: Pay attention to how your body feels after consuming artificial sweeteners. If you find they trigger cravings, you may be best off avoiding them.

DRINK WATER TO SPEED WEIGHT LOSS

A study by German researchers concluded that people who drink two 8-ounce glasses of water before a meal increased their rate of calorie burning by up to 30 percent about forty minutes later, and that rate stayed elevated for more than an hour. They concluded that drinking eight 8-ounce glasses of water could help burn an extra 35,000 calories a year! There are other benefits to drinking water. When you start dieting, your body loses fluid. If you don't get enough fluid, you're more prone to constipation and fluid retention, which can hide your actual weight loss. Dehydration can make you feel weak, and this may cause you to exercise less and eat more to compensate for the lack of energy. Most importantly, all biochemical reactions in the body, including digestion, take place in the presence of water. Adequate fluid intake allows your body to conduct its normal calorie burning process.

ACCELERATED WEIGHT LOSS MEAL PLANS

You should eat three meals a day, at the same times each day, as often as possible, plus a snack between breakfast and lunch, lunch and dinner, and after dinner, for a total of three per day. See chapter 6 for information on your daily calorie intake, and chapter 8 for the amount of physical exercise you should do each day.

The calories, carbs, and fat grams listed for the meal plans are estimates. They will vary depending on the product you choose. For example, the bread you choose may be lower in carbs and/or calories than the bread used in these plans, or the cheese you choose may be lower in calories and fat.

For you carb/gram counters out there, take note: I did not subtract the fiber from the total carbohydrate content in these meal plans. Many of the products in the My Favorite Foods section, pages 129–32, as well as foods in the meal plans, are high in fiber. As previously discussed, those of you are who are counting grams of carbohydrate may subtract the grams of fiber (if there are 5 grams or more per serving) from the total amount of carbohydrates. For example, two GG Scandinavian Crisp bread crackers contain 6 grams of carbs and 6 grams of fiber. The calculations in this plan count the crackers as 6 grams of carbs, whereas if you are counting grams of carbohydrate, you may count this product as 0 grams of carbohydrate.

The following meal plans contain approximately 1,100 calories a day, with 35 percent of the calories coming from carbs. These meal plans emphasize lower glycemic index carbs from vegetables, fruit, and whole grains. For the accelerated weight loss program, it is generally recommended that obese women with PCOS consume an 1,100 calorie diet.

Breakfast

For breakfast, target a calorie range from 140 to 210, grams of carbohydrate from 8 to 30, and grams of fat from 1 to 15. Initially, to accelerate weight loss and build momentum, you may want to focus on choices that are the lowest in calories, carbs, and fat.

1 cup 1% cottage cheese sprinkled with cinnamon. Add artificial sweetener, if desired.	160 cal, 8 gm carb, 2 gm fat
4 egg whites or egg substitutes 1 ounce soy cheese 1 slice whole grain bread	180 cal, 15 gm carb, 2 gm fat
omelet made with 1 egg, plus 3 whites ½ cup veggies cooked in cooking spray ½ grapefruit	190 cal, 16 gm carb, 5 gm fat
1 tablespoon almond butter 1 slice whole grain bread or 2 slices light whole grain bread or 80 calories high-fiber crackers	180 cal, 20 carb, 9 gm fat
tortilla roll-up: 1 ounce low-fat cheese 1 slice ham (½ ounce) 1 whole wheat tortilla	175 cal, 15 carb, 8 gm fat
1 tablespoon peanut butter on a small apple	180 cal, 19 gm carb, 9 gm fat
1 cup cooked oatmeal 4 chopped walnut halves artificial sweetener and cinnamon, if desired	210 cal, 25 carb, 7 gm fat
½ cup 1% cottage cheese ¾ cup blueberries	150 cal, 19 gm carb, 1 gm fat
8 ounces nonfat yogurt 2 tablespoons All-Bran (or another high-fiber cereal) 4 chopped walnut halves	170 cal, 18 gm carb, 5 gm fat

1 ounce low-fat cheese whole wheat English muffin	200 cal, 30 carb, 6 gm fat

2 ounces lox
1 tablespoon light cream cheese
1 mini whole wheat pita or
   80 calories of high fiber crackers
	200 cal, 15 gm carb,
	  11 gm fat

1 small orange 12 almonds	140 cal, 17 gm carb, 15 gm fat
3 scrambled egg whites or ½ cup egg substitutes 1 breakfast veggie sausage pattie 1 slice light whole grain bread 1 teaspoon light soft margarine	200 cal, 10 gm carb, 9 gm fat
2 poached eggs 1 cup cubed melon	210 cal, 15 gm carb, 10 gm fat
Fast-food breakfast out: McDonald's scrambled eggs	180 cal, 5 gm carb, 11 gm fat

LUNCH

For lunch, calories should range from 280 to 420, grams of carbohydrate from 3 to 25, and grams of fat from 5 to 30.

salmon, grilled, broiled, or
  poached, 4 ounces
1½ cup vegetables sautéed
  with 1 teaspoon olive oil
	335 cal, 12 gm carb,
	  17 gm fat

salad (3 cups salad greens),
  with 4 ounces grilled chicken
1 cup assorted vegetables
½ cup kidney beans
2 tablespoons light salad dressing
	360 cal, 21 gm carb,
	  9 gm fat

½ turkey (3 ounces) sandwich
  with lettuce, tomato, mustard
  on whole grain bread
cup of vegetable soup
	280 cal, 22 gm carb,
	  5 gm fat

tuna, water packed, 5 ounces 2 teaspoons low-fat mayo, chopped	315 cal, 18 gm carb, 9 gm fat

onions, and celery

80 calories of high-fiber crackers

salad greens

1 tablespoon light dressing

egg white omelet made with 3 egg whites	335 cal, 19 gm carb, 13 gm fat

1 ounce ham

1 ounce low-fat cheese

1 cup cooked mushrooms, spinach, and tomatoes

1 teaspoon oil in cooking

Pick one: 1 cup of soup (70 to 100 calories)
         80 calories of high-fiber crackers
         1 fruit (see fruit list)

turkey burger (ground turkey breasts), 5 ounces	340 cal, 13 gm carb, 10 gm fat

1 tablespoon ketchup

lettuce, tomato, sliced onion

1½ cups steamed vegetables

Tuna niçoise salad:	420 cal, 17 gm carb, 16 gm fat

4 ounces tuna, canned or fresh

3 ounces small boiled potato

2 egg whites, chopped

2 cups salad greens

2 tablespoons Italian dressing

Greek salad:	375 cal, 4 gm carb, 30 gm fat

3 cups greens, tomato slices

5 olives

3 ounces feta cheese

2 teaspoons oil, 2 tablespoons vinegar

Caesar salad with grilled chicken (6 ounces)	380 cal, 3 gm carb, 18 gm fat

3 cups greens

1 tablespoon Caesar dressing (on the side), add extra vinegar

no croutons, no extra Parmesan cheese

frozen, low-carb entrée, 300 calories or less	average: 370 cal, carbs, 13 gm fat

salad greens
2 tablespoons light dressing

Cheese melt:	325 cal, 25 gm carb, 12 gm fat
2 slices light whole grain bread	
2 ounces low-fat cheese	
tomato slices	
1 cup vegetable soup	

Cold pasta salad:	305 cal, 24 gm carb, 8 gm fat
½ cup cooked whole wheat pasta	
1½ cups assorted steamed veggies	
3 ounces tuna, shrimp, or grilled chicken strips	
1 tablespoon Italian dressing, plus 1 tablespoon balsamic vinegar	

3.75-ounce can sardines, oil packed, drained	346 cal, 23 gm carb, 12 gm fat
80 calories of high-fiber crackers	
75 calories of soup (read food label)	

1 cup lentil soup (or any non-cream soup of 150 calories or less, preferably one with beans, barley, vegetables, or lentils)	320 cal, 15 to 20 gm carb, 6 gm fat
3 ounces turkey breast or ⅔ cup 1% cottage cheese on greens with 50 calories of salad dressing	

Snacks

For snacks, calories should range from 60 to 150, grams of carbohydrate from 0 to 20, and grams of fat from 0 to 8.

½ ounce of nuts (see nut list)	80 cal, 3 gm carb, 8 gm fat
½ cup 1% cottage cheese and ½ cup blueberries	130 cal, 15 gm carb, 1 gm fat
2 teaspoons peanut butter and 60 calories of high-fiber crackers	150 cal, 13 gm carb, 6 gm fat
sugar-free yogurt (artificially	90 cal, 15 gm carb (varies),

sweetened) or low-carb yogurt, 6 to 8 ounces	0 gm fat
mini whole wheat pita and 1 teaspoon almond butter	115 cal, 15 gm carb, 5 gm fat
Baby Bel cheese and 1 small apple	110 cal, 15 gm carb, 3 gm fat
1 fruit	60 to 90 cal, 15 to 20 gm carb, 0 gm fat
1 ounce goat cheese, chopped tomato, basil on 50 calories of high-fiber crackers	125 cal, 9gm carb, 6 gm fat
1 tablespoon peanut butter on celery	100 cal, 2 gm carb, 8 gm fat
6 ounces nonfat plain yogurt (we recommend low-carb yogurt or Total 0% Fat Yogurt) with 2 teaspoons unsweetened cocoa or a splash of a flavored extract and added artificial sweetener, if desired	80 cal, 6 to 12 gm carb, 0 gm fat
3 GG Scandinavian crisp bread and ¾ ounce low-fat cheese (try Laughing Cow or Baby Bel)	90 to 110 cal, 9 gm carb, 4 to 7 gm fat
3-ounce can tuna, water packed, 1 teaspoon low-fat mayo, chopped celery and onions	130 cal, 0 gm carb, 3 gm fat
diet Jell-O, 4 ounces, with 2 table-spoons sugar-free whipped cream	25 cal, 3 gm carb, 0 gm fat
1 cup of vegetable soup	20 to 100 cal, 8 to 15 gm carb, minimal fat
3 ounces shrimp with 1 tablespoon cocktail sauce	110 cal, 5 gm carb, 2 gm fat
60 calories of high-fiber crackers with 2 tablespoons hummus	110 cal, 15 gm carb, 3 gm fat
one mini whole wheat pita with ½ ounce low-fat mozzarella cheese and 1 tablespoon tomato sauce	130 cal, 16 gm carb, 3 gm fat

Dinner

For dinner, calories should range from approximately 300 to 450, grams of carbs from 10 to 44, and grams of fat from 8 to 27.

6 ounces broiled scallops, with lemon   300 cal, 14 gm carb,
½ cup yellow peppers   8 gm fat
½ cup broccoli
½ cup carrots
1 small tomato, chopped
*Sauté all veggies with 1 teaspoon
   canola oil.*

5 oz sautéed swordfish, with   400 cal, 12 gm carb,
   chopped tomatoes and capers,   13 gm fat
   cooked in 1 teaspoon olive oil
roasted veggies (see recipe)

stir-fry with lean protein (see recipe)   425 cal, 33 gm carb,
½ cup brown rice   9 gm fat

Cajun pork chops (see recipe)   413 cal, 44 gm carb,
black bean salad (see recipe)   27 gm fat
1 cup steamed spinach with lemon

½ cup whole wheat pasta   425 cal, 25 gm carb,
4 ounces chicken   16 gm fat
sautéed veggies with 2 teaspoons olive
   oil, garlic, 1 small fresh tomato, ½ cup
   mushrooms, 1 cup fresh spinach
roast chicken, 6 ounces   405 cal, 10 gm carb,
gingered broccoli (see recipe)   11 gm fat
salad with 2 tablespoons light dressing

tomato sauce made with ¾ cup   350 cal, 22 gm carb,
   chopped tomatoes, fresh or canned,   17 gm fat
   1 teaspoon olive oil
3 ounces ground turkey breast
garlic, onions, seasoning
1½ cups cooked spaghetti squash
2 tablespoons Parmesan cheese
salad with 1 teaspoon olive oil,
   1 tablespoon vinegar

5 ounces broiled lean beef (lean beef has   450 cal, 15 gm carb,
   the words *loin* or *round* in the name: 19 gm fat
   top round, sirloin, eye round)
roasted veggies (see recipe)
sliced tomatoes and onions, 1 teaspoon
   olive oil, and unlimited vinegar

4 ounces shrimp	385 cal, 18 gm carb,
1 ounce feta cheese	19 gm fat
½ cup chopped tomatoes	
1 teaspoon olive oil	
8 large black olives	
1½ cups steamed broccoli	
veggie burger or 4 ounces turkey burger with 1 ounce low-fat cheese	410 cal, 23 gm carb, 15 gm fat (nutritional
2 slices whole wheat light bread or low-carb pita	content depends upon specific meal)
soup of 90 calories or less	
balsamic glazed chicken (see recipe)	465 cal, 32 gm carb,
½ cup wild rice	10 gm fat
1½ cups broccoli rabe sautéed with chopped garlic and 1 teaspoon olive oil	

Foods That Help Control Blood Sugar

There's a safe, natural food on the market that can help stabilize your blood sugar, yet it has no calories and tastes great. Sounds too good to be true? The latest research, conducted by Richard Anderson, Ph.D., at the Beltsville Human Research Nutrition Center in Maryland, shows that eating just half a teaspoon of cinnamon a day can do all that. If you find yourself overeating, the research suggests that your body may store fewer calories if you introduce cinnamon into your diet. It seems that cinnamon improves insulin activity in cells by increasing the rate at which they covert sugar to energy. Fat cells depend exclusively on sugar, so keeping your blood sugar levels stable deprives them of their one and only food source. Dr. Anderson's finding show that cinnamon can cut blood sugar levels by 20 to 30 percent.

Cinnamon is not the only food that helps fat cells behave more efficiently. In a study in which researchers gave the same amount of food to two groups of dieters, the group that got low-fat, high-calcium dairy foods lost up to 70 percent more weight. The research also shows that low-fat, high-calcium dairy foods can increase the loss of overall body fat by 64 percent, and help reduce belly fat by nearly 50 percent. This is great news for women with PCOS, who tend to gain excess weight around the abdomen.

turkey Marsala (see recipe) mashed cauliflower (see recipe) 1 cup of 70-calorie soup	400 cal, 24 gm carb, 12 gm fat (nutritional content depends on soup)
5 ounces broiled salmon (try brushing the fish with a little Dijon mustard before broiling) 3 ounces baked sweet potato, 1 teaspoon butter spray or light margarine 1 cup steamed green beans	455 cal, 22 gm carb, 18 gm fat
frozen dinner, preferably low-carb (300 calories or less) roasted asparagus (see recipe)	approximately 400 cal, 17 gm carb, 20 gm fat (calculations depend on frozen dinner)

RESTAURANT DINING

It's obvious that when you eat out, you often have little control over what exactly goes into the dish you order. But if you can't control the ingredients and preparation methods, at least you can select a restaurant that doesn't reek of burning fat.

CONTINENTAL

two appetizers: mixed green salad, 1 tablespoon dressing on the side and pick one: shrimp cocktail with 2 tablespoons cocktail sauce grilled shrimp tuna tartare grilled calamari	approximately 400 cal, 15 to 17 gm fat, minimal carb
steamed lobster, 6 ounces, with lemon steamed vegetable, 1½ cups salad with 1 tablespoon dressing	350 cal, 10 gm carb, 10 gm fat

filet mignon, 5 ounces (eat ½ portion)   400 cal, 10 gm carb,
steamed vegetable, 1½ cups   17 gm fat
salad with 1 tablespoon dressing

CHINESE

steamed protein (scallops, shrimp,   500 cal, 25 to 35 gm
    chicken, beef, tofu), approx 4 ounces,   carb, 10 to 17 gm fat
    and 2 cups of veggies
sauce on side, use 3 tablespoons
and
pick one: ½ cup brown rice
          2 steamed dumplings
          1 cup of soup

JAPANESE

If you choose to eat raw fish (for example, tuna tartare and sashimi) on occasion, do so at a reputable fish restaurant.

miso soup   495 cal, 15 gm carb,
½ order edamame   5 to 10 gm fat
sashimi, 5 pieces (tuna, yellowtail,
    and shrimp are lower in fat)
2 pieces sushi

MEXICAN

fajita, chicken, shrimp, or beef, 5 ounces   550 cal, 25 gm carb,
1 cup grilled onions and peppers   20 to 25 gm fat
one medium flour tortilla

Ask for minimal oil with preparation (assume 1 tablespoon).

THERMOGENIC EFFECT OF FOOD

Digestion takes energy, and your body uses food calories for energy. The amount of caloric energy it takes to digest and process the foods you eat is called is called *thermogenesis*. Different foods require different amounts of energy to digest, which means that the foods you choose can play a critical role in whether you gain or lose weight. Lean proteins such as fish, shrimp, and white-meat chicken have the highest thermogenic effect, with a full 30 percent of their calories being burned up during digestion. Conversely, simple carbohydrates such as cakes and bagels have a poor thermogenic effect, burning only 6 to 8 percent of their calories during digestion. High-fat foods have the poorest thermogenic effect, burning only 3 percent of their calories before going right to storage (often around your abdomen, if you have PCOS). White-meat chicken, fish, and seafood; high-fiber, low-starch green and white vegetables; egg whites; and high fiber are four thermogenic winners that speed up your metabolism, offer large volume, and put an end to out-of-control eating.

MEALS ON THE GO

While many of the big restaurant chains these days appear to be making serious efforts to provide healthy choices on their menus, some of the choices promoted as low in fat are high in unmentioned calories. Here are some choices that fit within the eating plan's guidelines at the time of this writing.

McDONALD'S

Grilled Chicken California Cobb Salad with Newman's Own Low-Fat Balsamic Vinaigrette Dressing	310 cal, 13 gm carb, 14 gm fat
Grilled Chicken Caesar Salad with Newman's Own Low-Fat Balsamic Vinaigrette Dressing (no croutons)	240 cal, 13 gm carb, 9 gm fat

BURGER KING

Fire Grilled Chicken Caesar Salad with
  Tomato Balsamic Vinaigrette Dressing
  (no croutons)

300 cal, 18 gm carb,
  16 gm fat

Fire Grilled Shrimp Garden Salad with
  Fat-Free Honey Mustard Dressing

255 cal, 28 gm carb,
  10 gm fat

WENDY'S

Mandarin Chicken Salad with roasted
  almonds (no rice noodles) and
  Low-Fat Creamy Ranch Dressing

400 cal, 27 gm carb,
  21 gm fat

(with no almonds)

270 cal, 23 gm carb,
  10 gm fat

SUBWAY

Grilled Chicken and Baby Spinach
  Salad with Kraft Fat-Free Italian
  Dressing and minestrone soup

265 cal, 25 gm carb,
  7 gm fat

BOSTON MARKET

Skinless Rotisserie Turkey Breast or
  ¼ white chicken, breast and wing,
  no skin, plus 2 side dishes of steamed
  veggies and sautéed spinach

290 cal, 8 gm carb,
  9 gm fat

APPLEBEE'S

Mesquite Chicken Salad

250 cal, gm carb n.a.,
  4 gm fat

Grilled Tilapia with Mango Salsa

320 cal, gm carb n.a.,
  6 gm fat

Teriyaki Shrimp Skewer

290 cal, gm carb n.a.,
  2 gm fat

MY FAVORITE FOODS

For any healthy food regimen to work, you have to enjoy what you are eating. If you don't, it won't be long before you find an acceptable excuse to eat something more to your liking. When you find healthful foods that you really enjoy, take note of them so that you can have them again. Here are some of my favorites:

LOW-FAT CHEESES

individually wrapped wedges of Laughing Cow Light	35 cal, 2 gm fat
¾ ounce Baby Bel individually wrapped portions	50 cal, 3 gm fat
1 ounce Cabot 75 % Reduced Fat Cheddar Cheese	60 cal, 3 gm fat
1 ounce Trader Joe's Fat-Free Sharp Cheddar	40 cal, 0 gm fat
1 ounce Alpine Lace Reduced Fat cheeses	70 cal, 5 gm fat
¾ ounce stick string cheese	varies 50 to 80 cal, 3 to 5 gm fat
1 slice Veggie Soy Cheese	40 cal, 2 gm fat

YOGURT AND COTTAGE CHEESE

Dannon Light 'n Fit Carb Control Strawberries and Cream Yogurt, 4 ounces	60 cal, 3 gm carb, 3 gm fat

Fage Total Greek 0% fat yogurt,   80 cal, 6 gm carb, 0 gm fat
5 ounces (Try it with flavored
extract or unsweetened cocoa
and artificial sweetener for an
unbelievably delicious low-calorie,
low-fat, and low-carb snack.)

4 ounces mini cottage cheese   80 cal, 6 gm carb, 2 gm fat

BREADS

Pepperidge Farm whole wheat,   60 cal, 8 gm carb,
low carb style bread, 1 slice   1.5 gm fat

Thomas Sahara 100% whole   70 cal, 13 gm carb, 1 gm fat
wheat mini pita

Sahara Carb Counting Pita,   90 cal, 20 gm carb, 2 gm fat
medium size

Arnold whole wheat light, 1 slice   40 cal, 9 gm carb, 0 gm fat

Van's Carb Manager Flax waffles,   100 cal, 10 gm carb,
1 waffle   7 gm fat

MEAT AND MEAT ALTERNATIVES

Oscar Mayer Fat-Free All Beef   40 cal, 3 gm carb, 0 gm fat
Frankfurters, 1 frank

Morningstar Farms, 2 veggie   80 cal, 3 gm carb, 3 gm fat
sausage links

Healthy Choice Roast Turkey or   60 cal, 3 gm carb,
Chicken packaged meats,   1.5 gm fat
4 slices

Morningstar Farms Tomato and   150 cal, 7 gm carb, 6 gm fat
Basil Pizza Burgers, 1 burger

WHOLE GRAIN CRACKERS

GG Scandinavian Crisp bread,   16 cal, 3 gm carb, 0 fat
per cracker

Kavili Hearty Rye, per cracker   35 cal, 8 gm carb, 0 gm fat

Ry-Vita (except Fruit Crunch),   35 cal, 8 gm carb, 0 fat
per cracker

Wasa Light Rye, per cracker   25 cal, 7 gm carb, 0 gm fat

| Ak-Mak 100% Whole Wheat Sesame Cracker, per cracker | 24 cal, 4 gm carb, 0.5 gm fat |
| Finn Crisp Caraway or Dark Rye, per cracker | 20 cal, 4 gm carb, 0 gm fat |

FATS

Smart Balance Spray, up to 5 one-second sprays	0 cal, 0 gm carb, 0 gm fat
I Can't Believe It's Not Butter! Spray, 5 sprays	0 cal, 0 gm carb, 0 gm fat
Pam Olive Oil Spray, ⅓ second spray	0 cal, 0 gm carb, 0 gm fat
Walden Farms Calorie Free Salad Dressing (in individual packets)	read label—nutritional content varies

VEGETABLE JUICE

| V8 Spicy Hot and Low Sodium Veggie Juice, 6 ounces | 35 cal, 8 gm carb, 0 gm fat |

SWEETS

Jeff's Diet Chocolate Soda	20 cal, 4 gm carb, 1.5 gm fat
Jell-O Sugar-Free, Fat-Free Chocolate Pudding, 4 ounces	35 cal, 8 gm carb, 0 gm fat
Kraft Fat-Free Cool Whip, 2 tablespoons	15 cal, 3 gm carb, 0 gm fat
Walden Farms Calorie-Free Chocolate Sauce, 2 tablespoons	0 cal, 0 gm carbs, 0 gm fat
Sugar-Free Jell-O, ½ cup	10 cal, 0 gm carb, 0 gm fat
Tofutti Chocolate Fudge Pops	30 cal, 6 gm carb, 0 gm fat
No Sugar Added Fudgsicle	40 cal, 10 gm carb, 1 gm fat
Weight Watchers chocolate mousse pop	60 cal, 14 gm carb, 0 gm fat

SOUPS

| Tabachnick French Onion Soup, 1 pouch | 50 cal, 11 gm carb, 0 gm fat |

Tabachnik Barley and Mushroom Soup, 1 pouch	80 cal, 16 gm carb, 5 gm fat
Campbell's Healthy Request Minestrone, 7.5 ounces	90 cal, 13 gm carb, 2 gm fat
Progresso Lentil, 9.5 ounces	140 cal, 25 gm carb, 4 gm fat
Amy's Organic Low-Fat Minestrone, 7 ounces	90 cal, 17 gm carb, 1.5 gm fat
Health Valley Mushroom Barley, 7.5 ounces	100 cal, 16 gm carb, 2 gm fat

FOR FLAVOR

These condiments have minimal calories, carbs, or fats:

Flavored vinegars, such as tarragon, balsamic, herb
Hot sauce
Salsa
Wine or chicken broth for cooking
Fresh ginger, garlic, and other herbs

HEALTHFUL SNACKS WHILE ON THE MOVE: NUTS

Nuts contain 160 to 200 calories per ounce, 13 to 20 grams of fat, and minimal carbs. Composed of both protein and fat, nuts are a great snack if you can control your portion size. They are filling and healthy. Different types of nuts (almonds, walnuts, pecans, pistachios, or peanuts) can improve your blood lipid levels and have a beneficial effect on cardiovascular risk. In addition, the Nurses' Health Study and Seventh Day Adventist Study have found lower body weights associated with increased nut consumption. While you can't lose weight on a nut-only diet, they may help you control your body weight. That said, if you can't limit yourself to a handful at a time, it's best to avoid them!

I recommend ½-ounce portions:

12 almonds	80 cal	7 walnut halves	95 cal
3 to 4 brazil nuts	95 cal	22 pistachios	80 cal
9 cashews	80 cal	14 peanuts	85 cal
10 hazelnuts	90 cal	¼ cup soy nuts	120 cal
5 to 6 macadamia nuts	100 cal	1 tablespoon sunflower	85 cal
10 pecan halves	100 cal	seeds (without shells)	

OPTICARBS

Try opticarbs for a group of low-glycemic carbohydrates that speed up weight loss while eliminating the cravings and hunger that sabotage so many diets. Opticarbs promote weight loss by controlling hunger and cravings, especially for high-glycemic carbohydrates, which can cause dramatic spikes in blood sugar; and by providing generous portions and superior nutrition for relatively few calories.

Opticarb foods include:

- High-calcium dairy, especially low- and non-fat yogurts, low-fat and fat-free cheeses, milk, and select dairy-based shakes.
- Green and white low-starch vegetables such as asparagus, broccoli, cucumber, cauliflower, and mushrooms. These vegetables are filling and full of fiber. High-fiber foods are important if you have PCOS, because they help slow the conversion of carbs into blood sugar, ensure healthy digestion and proper waste elimination, and control fat absorption. Fiber also binds to excess cholesterol and helps eliminate it from the body.
- GG Scandinavian Crisp bread is the only grain on the market that has zero "absorbed" carbs (the amount of carbs that have a tangible effect on your blood sugar), while supplying more fiber and fewer calories than other grains. If you have a history of abusing bread, they're the perfect substitute!

Opticarbs promote success at weight loss. Truly, they give you the carbs . . . without the consequences.

RECIPES

Here are some recipes to get you started on preparing the kind of healthful meals that will make a difference in your life. There are many suitable cookbooks to select recipes from and have adventures in preparing PCOS-friendly meals.

TURKEY MARSALA

2 turkey cutlets (7 ounces each)
2 tablespoons flour
cooking spray
2 teaspoons oil
1/2 pound mushrooms (button, shiitake, etc.), cleaned and sliced
1/3 cup Marsala wine
fresh ground pepper and salt to taste

Coat the cutlets with flour. Spray nonstick pan with vegetable cooking spray and sauté the cutlets about 2 minutes on each side. Remove. Add the 2 teaspoons oil to the same skillet and sauté the mushrooms until softened, about 4 minutes. Remove the mushrooms. Add the Marsala to the pan and cook for a few minutes over high heat. Add the turkey cutlets and mushrooms and heat for a minute or two. Add salt and pepper to taste.

2 servings   280 CAL, 8 GM CARB, 7 GM FAT PER SERVING

BALSAMIC GLAZED CHICKEN

2 chicken cutlets (6 ounces each), thinly sliced or pounded thin cooking
   spray
2 teaspoons vegetable oil
1 small red onion, chopped
1/2 cup chicken broth
2 to 3 tablespoons balsamic vinegar
1/4 teaspoon dried thyme
salt
freshly ground pepper

Cook the chicken cutlets in nonstick pan with cooking spray about 5 minutes on each side. Remove from the pan. Add 2 teaspoons of oil to the pan and sauté the onion for 5 minutes until soft. Add the chicken broth and balsamic vinegar and thyme; cook until the liquid reduces by a third. Add the chicken until it is heated. Season with salt and fresh pepper to taste.

2 servings   245 CAL, 3 GM CARB, 5 GM FAT PER SERVING

STIR-FRY RECIPE

5 ounces protein (chicken, shrimp, tofu, scallops, lean beef, or pork
   tenderloin)
4 cups assorted raw veggies (this will decrease to approximately
   2 1/2 cups when cooked):
         scallions, trimmed and thinly sliced
         thinly sliced cabbage
         shiitake or other mushrooms, sliced
         carrots, cut into thin slices
         broccoli flowerets
1 teaspoon sesame or vegetable oil
1 garlic clove, crushed
1 tablespoon light soy sauce
1/2 cup chicken broth (regular or low sodium)
2 tablespoons rice wine or dry sherry
optional: fresh grated ginger, 1 to 2 teaspoons
         hot mustard powder, 1/4 teaspoon
         crushed red pepper flakes, pinch

Stir frying is quick, so make sure you prepare the ingredients first. Slice the protein into thin strips. Cut the vegetables into julienne strips or bite-size pieces. Heat 1 teaspoon of oil in a nonstick pan. Add the protein and crushed garlic and cook for 3 minutes. Add the veggies; cook for 5 minutes or so, stirring frequently. Then add in the soy sauce, chicken broth, rice wine or dry sherry, and optional ingredients. Let this simmer for a few minutes until the vegetables are tender but not too soft. You may find that you want to adjust the ingredients the next time you make this recipe. Some people prefer it spicy, with more or less soy sauce, etc. Be creative—make it the way you like it!

1 serving   APPROXIMATELY 325 CAL, 12 GM CARB, 8 GM FAT, INCLUDING THE PROTEIN. OR, IF MADE JUST WITH VEGETABLES, APPROXIMATELY 110 CAL, 10 GM CARB, 4 GM FAT FOR 1½ CUPS. I RECOMMEND DOUBLING THIS RECIPE SO THAT YOU HAVE LEFTOVERS FOR ANOTHER MEAL.

ROASTED VEGGIES

1 red bell pepper and 1 yellow pepper, cored, seeded and cut into strips
1 cup fennel, sliced
2 red onions, peeled and cut into wedges
2 medium zucchini
8 ounces mushrooms, sliced
4 garlic cloves, peeled and thinly sliced
1 tablespoon balsamic vinegar
1 tablespoon olive oil
Pinch of dried or fresh herbs, if desired: oregano, thyme, rosemary, tarragon, parsley

Preheat oven to 425 degrees. In a large bowl, toss together all of the above ingredients. Place the vegetables in a baking dish or roasting pan; roast for 20 minutes or until tender and slightly browned, stirring several times. Add salt and freshly ground pepper as needed.

Approximately 3 servings   95 CAL, 8 GM CARB, 5 GM FAT PER 1 CUP SERVING

GINGERED BROCCOLI

1 tablespoon grated fresh ginger root
2 crushed garlic cloves
¼ cup rice vinegar
1 to 2 teaspoons Splenda
2 tablespoons light soy sauce
1 head broccoli

Combine the ginger, garlic, vinegar, Splenda, and soy sauce in a saucepan and bring to a boil. Wash the broccoli and cut into bite-size florets. Place in pan and cover. Steam for 5 minutes or until tender. Serve with some of the sauce.

60 CAL, 5 GM CARB PER 1 CUP SERVING

MASHED CAULIFLOWER

1 head cauliflower, washed and cut into bite-size pieces
*butter spray or 2 teaspoons light margarine (light margarines tend to
    have low levels of trans fats)*
1 to 2 tablespoons skim milk
salt and pepper to taste

Steam or microwave the cauliflower until tender. When cool, pat dry with paper towels to remove excess water. Add the butter spray or margarine and mash with a hand masher or blend in a food processor until smooth. Add 1 to 2 tablespoons of skim milk to thin, if needed. Add salt, pepper, and paprika to taste.

50 CAL, 6 GM CARB PER 1 CUP SERVING

CAJUN PORK CHOPS

¼ cup all-purpose flour
1 teaspoon Creole seasoning
½ teaspoon cayenne pepper
½ teaspoon black pepper
½ teaspoon garlic powder
1 teaspoon onion powder
1 tablespoon paprika
4 boneless pork chops (3 ounces of meat on each chop)
2 teaspoons canola oil

Whisk the flour and seasonings together in a pie pan or shallow bowl. Coat each pork chop. Heat the oil in a nonstick pan. Cook the pork chops approximately 7 minutes on each side over medium heat or until cooked through.

4 servings   205 CAL, 6 GM CARB, 9 GM FAT PER SERVING

BLACK BEAN SALAD

One 15-ounce can black beans, rinsed and drained
½ can (15-ounce) whole kernel corn, drained
4 green onions, chopped
1 jalapeño pepper, seeded and minced
½ red bell pepper, chopped and ½ green bell pepper, chopped
½ avocado, peeled, pitted, and diced
½ jar (4 ounces) pimentos
1½ tomatoes, seeded and chopped
½ cup chopped fresh cilantro
½ lime, juiced
¼ cup low-fat Italian salad dressing
¼ teaspoon garlic powder

Combine all the ingredients in a large bowl. Toss. Chill and serve.

6 servings   158 CAL, 32 GM CARB, 18 GM FAT

[8]

THE PCOS EXERCISE PROGRAM

A small amount of physical activity can have a relatively big impact on your health. In fact, the greatest health benefits from physical activity are derived not by the fit getting fitter, but by sedentary people who become just moderately active. In a twelve-year Swedish study, older people who exercised only once a week were 40 percent less likely to die than similar people who were totally sedentary. It seems that a little exercise goes a long way.

Exercise is the most effective way to keep from regaining the weight you lose on a healthy diet. This is not the only benefit of exercise, of course, but it is a persuasive argument for anyone who has successfully dieted and does not want to see her effort wasted, as so many women do when the weight comes back on. For women with PCOS, keeping their symptoms under control depends on not regaining the weight that they have lost.

In this chapter, I provide an exercise program divided into four levels. These levels are designed for women at different stages of fitness. As you become fitter, you progress from one level to another. You can select your own entry point at the appropriate level.

Level 1: First Steps. If you are sedentary, you may need to ease gently into very light or light activities and proceed from there. This two-week program helps you become consciously physically active, as opposed to being unthinkingly inactive.

Level 2: Walk for Fun. Once you are up and moving, it's time to go places. This six-week program starts out at a leisurely stroll and quickens the pace each week. At the end of this program you will already be fulfilling the minimum daily requirement of thirty minutes a day of moderate physical activity.

Level 3: Off and Running. This six-week program means what it says: On completing it, you can be assured that you will have achieved a reasonably healthy fitness level.

Level 4: Mixing It Up. You are now ready to participate in most low-impact exercise and sports. Don't allow yourself to become bored by a single activity. You'll find that this is a secret of long-term fitness.

Moderate activity consists of walking briskly at three or four miles per hour or another activity that causes your heart to beat at an equivalent rate. Most of us have only vague—and often highly inaccurate—notions of how active we are in the course of a day. The Centers for Disease Control and Prevention sent out a survey to get an idea of how everyday activities contributed to fitness levels. About a quarter of the respondents exercised on a regular basis. About half were not moderately active for the minimum recommended time of thirty minutes on at least five days a week. And about a quarter reported no regular moderate physical activity at all.

Some people live in areas without sidewalks, that are many miles from stores, and find they have to drive to shop and run errands, even if they would prefer to walk. Most of us don't have this excuse. In 2001, however, the average American over fifteen spent more than an hour a day behind a steering wheel. One simple way for a lot of us to become more active is to walk instead of drive to nearby destinations. Walking briskly for a mile burns about 100 calories. If you did that every day for a week, you would burn 700 calories. In a year, you would burn at least 35,000 calories. Let's do some weight-loss math. For every 3,500 calories burned, you lose one pound, so walking instead of driving to the store could add up to ten pounds a year.

It sounds easy. What's the catch?

The catch is that habits are harder to break than most people realize. We strongly resist even small changes in our lifestyles, even when they make us feel better almost immediately. We formed most of our habits in childhood and adolescence. A few of us formed healthful eating and exercise habits then and are currently reaping the rewards. A few of us inherited genes that seem to protect us from harm, no matter how we live or what we do. Most of us, unfortunately, don't have ingrained healthy habits or all-protective genes. We need to look more closely at how we live and making some changes for the better. This is what the PCOS exercise program enables you to do, with as little effort and as much pleasure as possible.

LAURA'S STORY

Laura's new house was only ten minutes from the train station, so she decided to commute by rail to her job in Manhattan after twenty years of driving. Although her trip involved a subway ride after her commuter train arrived at Grand Central, she no longer had to put up with traffic-clogged highways and high city garage fees. As she carried her briefcase up and down ramps and staircases in the rush hour crowds, Laura at first often became winded. With time, the physical effort took less out of her. From the beginning, she had noticed that people on public transportation were noticeably thinner than people who drove to work in the city. New York City was hardly a health spa, but she had to say she was feeling great and was gradually losing weight after her workday treks through the Big Apple's subterranean passageways.

Laura's account fits in with the results of a San Diego study in which 65 percent of people who lived in less walkable areas (no sidewalks, far from stores) were overweight, in comparison with 35 percent of people in walkable city neighborhoods. One researcher observed that these people were not more active because they wanted to be. They often *had* to walk.

REVISED FEDERAL GUIDELINES

Revised guidelines released on January 12, 2005, by the departments of Agriculture and Health and Human Services emphasize that weight loss depends on caloric intake and regular exercise, rather than avoiding specific foods. While previous guidelines recommended thirty minutes of moderate exercise on most days of the week, the new guidelines stress that this amount of activity is a minimum rather than a desirable amount. Instead, the new guidelines recommend the following:

Minimum physical activity	30 minutes a day of moderate exercise
To keep from gaining weight	60 minutes a day of moderate to vigorous exercise
To lose weight	60 to 90 minutes a day of moderate to vigorous exercise

To many people the idea of an hour of exercise a day seems an almost impossible demand. Even if you are willing, who has the time? My suggestion is to focus on finding activities you truly enjoy doing. You'll be amazed how motivated you become to find time for things you really love to do. That's exactly where this exercise program takes you—at level 4, you pick and choose what you feel like doing.

BURNING CALORIES

Besides helping to prevent weight gain, exercise makes your body function better and builds muscles. Muscle tissue has a high metabolic rate, burning calories instead of storing them. Every pound of muscle that you develop burns an extra thirty-five to fifty calories a day. On a medical level, physical activity, regardless of its intensity, lowers your risk for diabetes and cardiovascular disease, as well as improves high blood pressure, insulin sensitivity, blood sugar control, and blood lipid levels.

When you burn calories through exercise, expect your body to fight back. We still have the bodies of our hunter-gatherer ancestors, who gorged themselves in times of plenty and spent the rest of the time on the brink of starvation. Like theirs, our bodies are designed to conserve the fuel we have stored in the form of fat. As you exercise, if you don't eat enough food to replenish the calories you are burning, your body tries to conserve energy by becoming more efficient. The 100 calories you burn by running one mile today may be only 90 calories for the same distance tomorrow. This helped our ancestors survive, but acts as an obstacle to your weight loss agenda.

Small, everyday activities that burn calories add up over time to make a real difference. For example, walking up stairs at your workplace (if you can do so) instead of taking the elevator burns more than 100 calories a day, which could add up to a weight loss of more than ten pounds a year. Look for such possible mini activities during the course of your day.

Remember, too, that it takes very little food to cancel out

the benefits of a lot of exercise. A single cookie or two apples can cancel out the 300 calories you burned by running for forty-five minutes.

The following are the approximate number of calories a 150-pound woman would burn if she continued the activity for half an hour.

Activity	Calories Burned in 30 Minutes
Jogging	340
Climbing stairs	305
Tennis	275
Heavy lifting	275
Weightlifting	235
Bicycling	220
Aerobics	170
Gardening	170
Walking briskly	150
Shopping	120
Housework	120
Walking around	85
Preparing a meal	75
Sedentary deskwork	50
Watching TV	35

You can check the number of calories burned in various activities at http://www.caloriecontrol.org/exercalc.html.

FITNESS VERSUS WEIGHT LOSS

Fitness is a boon, regardless of your weight. This was shown in a four-year study on the cardiovascular health of 906 women. More than 75 percent of the women were overweight, 70 percent had low fitness levels, and almost 40 percent already had coronary artery disease. Those with low fitness levels were almost 50 percent more likely to have cardiovascular trouble, and fit, overweight women had better outcomes than unfit, thin women.

While fitness plays a great role in cardiac health, weight loss may be more important in diabetes. We know that in comparison with women of normal weight, overweight women are three times as likely to develop type 2 diabetes, and obese women are nine times as likely, and that these risk levels are little affected by the fitness levels of the women. However, according to Dr. Gerald M. Reaven, insulin resistance is related to physical fitness. He regards lack of fitness as important as obesity in predicting insulin sensitivity.

It can be difficult, of course, to separate the benefits of fitness and weight loss, because the two so often accompany each other. Physical activity helps you lose weight, and when you lose weight, physical activity keeps you from regaining it. That's the happy relationship between the two that you need to keep in mind. Additionally, as you become fitter, you start to feel better, both physically and emotionally.

STARTING THE PCOS EXERCISE PROGRAM

As mentioned earlier, the program has four levels. Read through the program and decide where you're going to start. If you were too ambitious—or not ambitious enough—your body will tell you and you can either take a step back or ramp things up with the next level. You choose an entry point in one of the levels. Go backward in weeks or levels if the activity proves too hard, or forward if it is too easy. Rely on your judgment. Don't rush things. Repeat a week when you feel the need for it. Listen to your body.

The chart below is for general reference. The intensity of effort that you put into a light activity can raise it to a moderate one, or make a moderate activity vigorous.

Very Light Activity	Light Activity	Moderate Activity	Vigorous Activity
Cooking	Housework	Gardening	Tennis
Yard work	Golf	Bicycling	Basketball
Ironing	Much non-sedentary, indoor work	Brisk walking	Running
Walking around	Childcare on good days	Swimming	Heavy lifting
Shopping	Much volunteer work	Jogging	Weight lifting
		Low-impact aerobics	Climbing stairs

LEVEL 1: FIRST STEPS

Vera went from tennis in her twenties, to hiking in her thirties, to shopping in her forties, to finding her car in her fifties. Sometimes a week passed without her ever walking a hundred yards at a time. She had PCOS and, needless to say, a weight problem. You could call Vera highly sedentary, and I have no problem in placing her at Level 1 in our exercise program.

Researchers have estimated that for sedentary people, basic metabolic processes account for 80 percent of the energy burned, with physical activity accounting for only 10 percent. Digestion of food accounts for the final 10 percent. As you know, additional calories not burned for energy are stored in the body, often as body fat. Thus, for very inactive people, the kind of food they eat becomes very important. For them, surplus calories from high-calorie foods go directly to storage. The more active you are, the less you need to worry about the calorie content of the foods you eat.

The average person takes about 6,000 steps a day, which amounts to three miles. Walking another 2,000 steps (an extra mile) would make a positive difference in the health of most of these people. Small changes like this can be an ideal way for previously inactive people to embark on a more active lifestyle. It's too soon for them to wonder what exercises might best suit them—their primary goal is to simply to make time for some form of exercise on their daily agenda. It almost goes without saying that if you are not sure whether you are active, you are almost certainly inactive.

People who have been nearly totally sedentary for years may read, see, or hear something that inspires them to lead a more active life from that moment onward. Rather than consider what kind of low-impact activity might best suit their unfit condition, they may decide to run a mile or attempt to lift sixty pounds. Fortunately for most, they're confronted with reality before they hurt themselves. I believe in taking things very gradually at first. In fact, if you are sedentary, I recommend that during the two weeks that you are at this level, and before you progress to Level 2, have your physician advise you on the kinds of physical activity that are safest for you.

| Week 1 | 30 minutes/day | Engage in very light or light physical activities |
| Week 2 | 60 minutes/day | Engage in light physical activity |

The thirty or sixty minutes required can be divided into shorter periods, and the very light or light physical activities can be as various as you wish. The point is to be active without overdoing it.

LEVEL 2: WALK FOR FUN

Roni is overweight and has PCOS. I once considered her very sedentary for a thirty-two-year-old, but after following the program for two weeks she already feels more flexible, something she notices every time she gets up from an armchair or in and out of her car.

While walking, wear loose-fitting clothes and comfortable shoes or sneakers. Stay in safe, well-traveled areas, and don't assume that everyone outdoors in the early morning is there for fresh air. Avoid unpleasantly hot times of the day by walking earlier or later.

The fact that this is a six-week program does not mean that you must complete it in six weeks. If you miss a few days in any particular week, repeat that week again. Also, if for any reason you feel unready for the next step, there is no need to push yourself to the next level. Simply repeat the week at which you are comfortable, and continue to do so until you are ready to move on.

You can substitute any similar activity for walking briskly. Swimming is a popular alternative.

Many women find that sharing an activity with a friend—pets included—makes the whole enterprise a lot more fun. Plus, you're more motivated to stick with it—your friend's expecting you!

	Walk	Walk Briskly	Walk	Total Time
Week 1	5 minutes	5 minutes	5 minutes	15 minutes/day
Week 2	5 minutes	10 minutes	5 minutes	20 minutes/day
Week 3	5 minutes	15 minutes	5 minutes	25 minutes/day
Week 4	5 minutes	20 minutes	5 minutes	30 minutes/day
Week 5	5 minutes	25 minutes	5 minutes	35 minutes/day
Week 6	5 minutes	30 minutes	5 minutes	40 minutes/day

LEVEL 3: OFF AND RUNNING

Weighing 204 pounds at age 24 and just having been diagnosed with PCOS, Julie started the program at Level 2 and repeated the week to get used to everyday activity before trying anything more strenuous. She now feels she should perhaps have started at Level 3. Julie has plenty of energy but is not the most patient person. Is she ready to structure a new lifestyle? Will she stay with the program, or discard it for some new thing? Repeating the first week at Level 2 is a good sign that she's committed to doing this for good. If she goes, she can always come back. For now, she is at an enthusiastic Level 3.

It's always a good idea to mention to your doctor that you will be participating in more vigorous activities. Even if you have cardiovascular problems, he or she will probably welcome the news.

Wear sneakers and a track suit in colder weather or a T-shirt and shorts in warmer weather. You don't need to spend lots of money on the latest gear to get fit, but well-fitting clothes made of moisture-wicking material are a great way to pat yourself on the back for sticking with the program.

If you become too flushed or out of breath, stop until you recover and then go home. Don't push yourself to finish that day—in fact, skip the next day if you do not feel well. Never try to run through the pain.

This is a six-week program, but my advice for Level 2 applies here, too: Repeat weeks when you feel you're not ready to go on to the next. You can also swim rather than jog, if you prefer. (*Julie update:* She completed the program, lost more than fifteen pounds, and noted a real improvement in her PCOS symptoms.)

	Walk & Stretch	Slow Jog	Walk	Full Jog	Walk & Stretch	Total Time
Week 1	5 minutes	1 minute	5 minutes	1 minute	5 minutes	17 minutes/day
Week 2	5 minutes	3 minutes	5 minutes	1 minute	5 minutes	19 minutes/day
Week 3	5 minutes	5 minutes	5 minutes	3 minutes	5 minutes	23 minutes/day
Week 4	5 minutes	3 minutes	5 minutes	5 minutes	5 minutes	23 minutes/day
Week 5	5 minutes	2 minutes	5 minutes	10 minutes	5 minutes	27 minutes/day
Week 6	5 minutes	5 minutes	2 minutes	15 minutes	5 minutes	32 minutes/day

LEVEL 4: MIXING IT UP

It took Martha nine weeks to arrive at Level 4. Like most of us, between work and family there are too many demands on her time. But she never gave up. At thirty-six, she does not allow her PCOS, type 2 diabetes, or high blood pressure to limit her life. A teacher, she rarely misses a day of school, even when she feels truly awful. Reaching Level 4 for her is a real achievement and gives her confidence that she can do and achieve whatever she wants.

Don't get stuck feeling you have to do the same thing day after day. Walk or jog when you feel like it, or try a low-impact exercise or sport. Experiment until you find several things that you really enjoy. Then follow your fancy. After work and on weekends, ask friends if you can tag along on their favorite outings. Join clubs or teams on a trial basis. Word of mouth, free newspapers, and the Internet are your best sources of information on what is happening locally. Stores that sell shoes and fitness or sports equipment can be sources of info for clubs and teams. A friend who recently bought a pair of running shoes told me that the clerk asked her if she wanted her name on an e-mail list to receive announcements of local programs and events.

I think it's a good idea to take a few classes before attempting to work out at home, with or without videotapes. Alignment is important in many of these activities, and with an instructor you can do things right from the very beginning.

There are no specific daily guidelines for the multiple activities at this level. My only concern is that you don't overexert or overtire yourself. Stop the activity if you feel that you are becoming too hot or winded. Don't fixate on one activity or do any one thing for hours on end. Here are some popular activities that you may find of interest.

Functional training. This popular new trend combines a cardiovascular workout with rehab techniques that help prepare you for small, unexpected challenges such as uneven or icy sidewalks, running for a bus, or reaching at an awkward angle. The exercises focus on your body's core abdominal and spinal muscles and on improving your reaction speed, agility, and balance. Weaving at speed between plastic cones, stepping quickly over inches-high hurdles, muscle toning with exercise balls, and working out on drill mats are part of the hour-long classes.

Yoga. Finding a good teacher is more important than finding the kind of yoga that might best suit you. A good teacher will inquire about neck, lower back, or knee problems that can be aggravated over time by certain yoga poses or asanas, as most teachers call them. He or she may offer modifications or alternative poses.

Pilates. As with yoga, finding a good teacher is the most important thing. This technique helps build abdominal and back muscles.

Tai chi. A good teacher is also essential in this activity, to make sure you are doing the movements correctly. Both tai chi and yoga are wonderful for restoring body flexibility, loss of which is often one of the most evident signs of aging.

Exercise ball. If you prefer to work out at home, an exercise ball that costs $20 to $40 may be just right for you. Most exercises involve sitting or lying facedown or faceup on the ball. Many of the exercises are those commonly performed on the floor, but when you do them on a ball, its instability forces you to use far more muscles than you would if you were doing the same exercises on a floor mat—mostly abdominal muscles.

Weight lifting. It's a myth that women who lift weights develop muscles in their arms and legs like a man's. Women who avoid the weight room for this reason miss out on a great way to prevent osteoporosis, as well as build shapely, feminine muscle tissue. Muscle tissue burns calories even when you are at rest.

A WORD OF CAUTION

If you worry about injury while exercising, see your doctor before rather than afterward. If you exercise to excess, you can hurt yourself. Throwing yourself into strenuous activities that you are not conditioned for makes injury not only possible but likely. It is said that vigorous exercise triggers up to 17 percent of sudden cardiac deaths in the United States, which amounts to tens of thousand of deaths a year. In this case, you can do too much of a good thing.

At what kinds of exercise do women most often hurt themselves? The following emergency room admission data were collected by the Sports Medicine Center at the University of Rochester.

All Females	Percent of Total Injuries	Women 45 or Older	Percent of Total Injuries
Bicycling	13	Exercise	23
Basketball	9	Bicycling	14
Playground	9	Horseback	7
Exercise	8	Golf	4
Gymnastics	6	Gymnastics	4
Soccer	5	Swimming	4

Respect your limitations. Age may be one of them. Your present state of fitness is one. A chronic or temporary illness may be another. For example, women with diabetes over the age of thirty-five to forty should undergo stress testing before participating in moderate or more physical activity. Much of this is common sense.

You don't drive your car at a hundred miles per hour, so don't put your foot too heavily on the gas when driving your body. You're in this for the long haul, so pace yourself. Start and progress slowly and rest assured that exercise prolongs far more lives than it cuts short.

[9]

GETTING PREGNANT

If you want to start a family, I've got good news: Your likelihood of conceiving and having a healthy baby, in spite of PCOS, is very high. I start this chapter with this encouraging message because it is so easily lost in a discussion of the complicated forces at work in PCOS. It's possible you'll become pregnant without doing anything for your health. But if you lose some weight, your chances of conceiving are much greater. If you're carrying extra pounds, weight loss is healthy and a good idea, in any case. It's certainly the best way to start. If weight loss doesn't work, fertility drugs very likely will. We will look at two frequently prescribed drugs in this chapter, one of which I recommend over the other, although there are times when I suggest using them in combination.

Carrying your unborn child inside your body puts extra physical stress on your biological systems. Any system already out of balance may be made more so by this added stress. It makes sense, therefore, to have your body in the best working order possible before becoming pregnant. A woman with PCOS, besides often having trouble in conceiving, has more difficulty in getting her body into a reasonably healthy condition. Although taking steps to improve your health before a pregnancy may not be easy to achieve, it can make a big difference in your future well-being and your child's.

If you have been diagnosed with PCOS and want to conceive, I strongly recommend:

- Losing about 10 percent of your body weight and engaging in brisk activity for at least half an hour each day. The weight loss and exercise will help lower high blood pressure and high insulin and male hormone levels.
- Having a complete physical checkup, including a full array of lab tests. Discuss any abnormal lab test results with your doctor in light of your plans for bearing a child.
- Discussing with your doctor your impaired glucose tolerance or type 2 diabetes status. I'll address this in the type 2 diabetes section in chapter 10.
- Taking prenatal vitamins prescribed by your gynecologist.

Once you are pregnant, your obstetrician may decide to supplement you with progesterone if your hormone levels are short of what's needed to maintain a healthy pregnancy.

ON CONCEIVING

There is a relatively short time in each menstrual cycle when an egg can be fertilized by sperm. Normal women with regular cycles often have trouble conceiving simply because of poor timing and are usually advised to keep trying. For women with irregular cycles, timing is even more problematic. But fertility problems are more than a matter of timing for many women with PCOS, because even when they have regular menstrual cycles, they often do not ovulate.

When they do ovulate, women with PCOS can conceive without any medical assistance, and often do. (About a quarter of women with PCOS have regular cycles, and some conceive without medication.) Individuals vary greatly in their symptoms—there are women with regular cycles who may or may not ovulate, those with irregular cycles who may ovulate on occasion, and those who almost never have a cycle or ovulate.

Don't jump to the conclusion that PCOS is responsible for your fertility problem. Adhesions, endometriosis, uterine fibroids, fallopian tube problems, or cervical mucus disturbances could present physical obstacles to conception. A number of systemic or hormonal disturbances, such as thyroid disease, prolactin secreting disorders, excessive weight, pituitary and adrenal disorders, genito-urinary disease, or infections (for example, pelvic inflammatory disease) may be the primary cause of the infertility. And, of course, your partner may have issues of his own.

Before settling on PCOS as the cause of infertility, the other possible causes have to be eliminated. Once that is done, if you have irregular or infrequent periods, with sometimes heavy bleeding, PCOS is likely to be responsible, although this is not a diagnosis you can make yourself. A competent gynecologist is important in excluding local gynecological diseases or barriers to achieving pregnancy. An ultrasound of your ovaries and uterus is one of many tests that will help identify the problem.

OVULATION TESTS

Clearly you cannot become pregnant unless you ovulate. For a woman with PCOS, having menstrual cycles is no guarantee that she is ovulating. The following three ovulation tests are popular. I recommend using more than one for reasons I'll explain below.

Home kits. Home kits do not measure ovulation itself but the luteinizing hormone (LH) surge that precedes the release of the egg from the follicle. The over-the-counter kits usually consist of five test sticks to measure the LH level in your urine. If a test line on the stick becomes darker than a control line, you are having an LH surge. If the test line stays lighter than the control line, you are not—and should try again the next day with a new test stick.

For a woman with regular cycles, the arrival of an LH surge means that she is likely to ovulate in the next twenty-four hours. Unfortunately, things are not so simple for women with PCOS, whose high levels of LH are not necessarily a precursor to ovulation. Either way, though, this is the best time to try to conceive—it can't hurt!

Basal body temperature. Ovulation causes your body temperature to rise by 0.3 to 0.5 degrees Fahrenheit (0.2 degrees Centigrade) or higher, due to a higher progesterone level. Your body remains at this slightly higher temperature until your next period. The challenge is to detect this small temperature rise.

One of the best ways of doing so is to take your temperature at the same time each morning, preferably before you get out of bed. For reliability, you really do need to take the reading at the same time each day. A difference of even a half hour can affect the reading. Stress, lack of sleep, an extra glass of wine consumed the night before, a cold, or medication can also affect your temperature reading.

Most women take their own temperature by mouth, with either a mercury or digital thermometer. Taking an oral temperature with a digital thermometer is the most convenient. You can get a special chart from your doctor on which to record your daily temperature readings.

By the time you capture the increase in your body temperature on paper, it may be too late for you to conceive in this cycle.

But for most women with PCOS, the fact that ovulation took place at all is good news in itself.

Progesterone blood level. This lab test on a blood sample taken in your doctor's office during days 21 to 23 of your cycle measures your progesterone level. If you ovulated, your progesterone level will be elevated. The result of this test is a more reliable indicator of ovulation than a positive home kit test result or a rise in basal body temperatures.

PELVIC PAIN THERAPY

Although pelvic pain is not often mentioned in medical journal articles as a common PCOS symptom, my experience suggests that at least one in ten women with PCOS suffers from it. Ovarian discomfort and small follicle cyst ruptures, sometimes after sexual activity, are probably responsible. These occur more dramatically in women prone to cystic ovarian adenomas, dermoid cysts, and recurrent large follicular or corpus luteum cysts. In rare instances, major bleeding emergencies can occur, requiring instant medical attention and surgery. Suppressive therapy with an oral contraceptive is indicated, and such a woman's progress needs to be followed by an experienced gynecologist, with frequent examinations and ultrasound follow-ups.

BEFORE TRYING INFERTILITY DRUGS

Weight loss alone is sufficient to enable some women with PCOS to ovulate and subsequently become pregnant. Before resorting to medications, first try a weight loss program. The one I recommend to my patients is described in detail in chapters 6 and 7. In any case, it's a good idea to establish healthy eating and exercise habits. Truly that may be all you need.

If that doesn't work, two drugs have been very successful in enabling women with PCOS to ovulate: metformin and clomiphene citrate. Let's look at both.

Metformin

Metformin (brand name Glucophage) was approved by the FDA in 1994 for use in the management of type 2 diabetes. It lowers your blood sugar level by slowing the liver's release of stored glucose and lowers insulin resistance in muscle tissue. Metformin also helps lower LDL cholesterol levels somewhat and does not cause hypoglycemia, because it does not increase insulin secretion. It also frequently reduces testosterone levels and may result in weight loss. Metformin is the most widely used oral agent in the treatment of adults with type 2 diabetes. Millions of Americans take it, and most physicians are familiar with it.

Metformin can trigger a series of events that lead to more regular menstrual cycles and ovulation. Having PCOS, however, does not automatically mean you should be using this drug. Some prominent experts prefer other treatment strategies. For example, metformin may not be the initial drug of choice for women suffering from PCOS-related skin and hair symptoms but who are not obese and have regular ovulatory cycles.

The side effects of metformin can appear early, but frequently diminish after six to eight weeks of use. They include bloating, nausea, vomiting, flatulence, and diarrhea. Every person taking the drug reacts differently. Some women (in my experience, fewer than 5 percent) are unable to tolerate it at all, while others have few if any side effects.

Before starting metformin treatment, you need a pelvic ultrasound examination, and your doctor will probably prescribe progestin to initiate a menstrual cycle—often 10 mg Provera daily for seven to ten days, or a 200 mg Prometrium capsule in the evening for seven to ten days. You may have heavy bleeding following this.

I then start patients on a 500 mg tablet of metformin taken with dinner for ten to fourteen days. If there are minimal or no side effects, we add a second 500 mg tablet at breakfast time. Side effects become less frequent as your body becomes accustomed to the drug, and the dosage is gradually increased, depending on symptoms, to 2,000 mg daily, split between breakfast and dinner doses. A new oral liquid form of metformin has been useful in some cases. An overly rapid increase in dosage is a major cause of women being unable to tolerate metformin, so be patient.

After two to three months of treatment, you may notice more regular cycles. You can also test whether you have ovulated with home test kits, basal body temperature curves, and, most useful, your progesterone blood level on days 21 to 23 of your cycle.

If tests indicate that you did not ovulate on a divided dosage of 2,000 mg of metformin a day over three to six months, your next step is to add clomiphene citrate on days 5 to 9 of your next cycle. Most women with PCOS ovulate on this regimen and often become pregnant during the next few months. Metformin and clomiphene citrate together help 75 to 80 percent of women with PCOS ovulate, which is greater than using metformin alone. It's your gynecologist's responsibility to evaluate you during clomiphene treatment, since on occasion it may cause significant enlargement of the ovaries and pelvic pain. An increase in multiple births has been reported with clomiphene citrate, but this has not been reported with metformin alone.

Although metformin has been shown not to affect the fetus, I recommend that you stop the drug once your pregnancy is confirmed.

Metformin reduces insulin resistance, decreases fatty liver formation, reduces risk factors for cardiovascular disease and clotting, and improves to some extent blood lipid levels. Metformin may protect the heart, reduce high blood pressure, and lower male hormone levels. It probably delays the development of type 2 diabetes. It helps both overweight and normal-weight women with PCOS to achieve ovulation. Some experts believe that many of the benefits attributed to metformin may in fact be due to the weight loss that occurs in a number of women taking the drug. To some extent, this may be true. What is known, however, is that the beneficial effects occur in most studies, despite an absence of weight loss during administration of the drug.

I usually make the following recommendations to my patients who take metformin:

To avoid hypoglycemia, you should eat a somewhat reduced carbohydrate diet consisting of six small meals a day. Hypoglycemia is not caused by metformin, but perhaps by an overly strict low-carbohydrate diet. The mid-afternoon hours are times when insulin-resistant women with PCOS may feel uncomfortable, fatigued, and less able to concentrate, so plan to snack on a combination of complex sugars and proteins. I often recommend a snack of a green apple with low-carb peanut butter.

Avoid alcohol. I highly recommend that you avoid alcohol while on metformin therapy.

Cautions. If, for some reason, you need a CT scan—more specifically, an intravenous iodine contrast diagnostic CT scan—

CONTROLLING WEIGHT WITH METFORMIN

Diet and exercise are difficult to adhere to. When women with PCOS cannot achieve a 5 to 7 percent loss of body weight through diet and exercise as their first course of treatment, their doctors may consider the use of insulin sensitizers, particularly for women with moderate to severe insulin resistance or features of the insulin resistance syndrome. The drugs Actos and Avandia, despite their ability to lessen insulin resistance, can promote weight gain and thus make PCOS symptoms worse. Metformin, a member of a different family of drugs, the biguanides, frequently promotes or "triggers" weight loss as well as reduces insulin resistance. It helps many women lose weight through loss of appetite, which is a great relief to women with PCOS who can suffer sugar cravings, an out-of-control appetite, and mood swings. Often, long before reaching the optimum daily 2,000 mg dosage, women often feel its ameliorating effects on their appetites. Some women lose weight, notice a decrease in appetite and sugar cravings, and fewer hypoglycemic symptoms after eating at half that dose. These positive signs can indicate a reduction in insulin level and provide a substantial emotional and physiological boost.

stop taking metformin the day before, the day of the test, and the morning after. This prevents any possible hazardous elevation of the metformin blood level due to the effect of iodine on your kidneys and the very rare and serious complication of lactic acidosis.

Have your creatinine level checked at least every three to six months. Any increase is a warning that your kidneys are being overworked. If it approaches 1.4 mg percent, stop taking metformin. If you have any pre-existing kidney disease, you should use metformin with caution, if at all.

CLOMIPHENE CITRATE

Clomiphene citrate (brand names Clomid and Serophene) can be used alone for infertility therapy or in combination with metformin, as discussed above. Clomiphene citrate is not a steroid hormone or an insulin sensitizer. It is a weak estrogen that binds to the hypothalamic and pituitary estrogen receptors, making them blind to the estrogens that are circulating in the blood. This allows the pituitary gland to secrete more LH and FSH, stimulating the ovaries and encouraging follicle development that leads to ovulation.

Your physician can use your pituitary FSH and LH blood levels as a guide to your chances of responding to clomiphene citrate. A minority of women with PCOS may have low levels of LH, FSH, and estradiol due to lack of menstrual bleeding, even after taking progestin for seven days. They may not respond to clomiphene citrate treatment. These women appear to have reduced activity of the hypothalamic and pituitary glands, a state that may be caused by a very lean BMI of 20 or less, malnutrition, eating disorders, excessive stress, or emotional problems. Obviously it's important to address these issues, and professionals can help.

Before you start taking clomiphene citrate, you need a blood b-hCG test to make sure that you are not already pregnant. The standard starting dose of clomiphene citrate is 50 mg (1 tablet) a day for 5 days, from days 5 to 9 (occasionally days 3 to 7) of your menstrual cycle, after a natural or progestin-induced menstrual flow. The majority of women with PCOS need to take progestin to trigger a menstrual cycle. About 50 percent of patients conceive at the 50 mg dose, while another 20 percent achieve pregnancy with a 100 mg dose of clomiphene citrate. If no ovulation occurs at the 50 mg dosage, the daily dose can be upped progressively to a maximum of 200 to 250 mg for up to 3 months.

If a woman is responsive to clomiphene citrate, she is likely to be so within three or four cycles. The surge of ovulation usually occurs on cycle days 16 to 17, when clomiphene citrate is used from days 5 to 9 of the cycle. However, 5 to 12 days may pass after the last day of clomiphene citrate treatment before the ovulatory surge. Since the majority of patients who respond to clomiphene citrate get pregnant in the first three months, beyond that point you and your doctor should look for other causes of infertility.

Cautions. Often the length of your menstrual cycle will increase slightly with clomiphene citrate. The drug increases a woman's chance of having twins by 8 to 10 percent, and of having triplets by about 1 percent. The drug sometimes causes increased cervical mucus that reduces your chances of conceiving—it can literally get in the way.

The potential for the development of ovarian cancer in women treated with clomiphene citrate and gonadotropins has been the focus of several studies. There are none as yet that confirm an increased incidence of ovarian cancer in a large number of such women. It is prudent, however, to limit treatment to no more than one year.

Because clomiphene citrate stays in the blood for at least three to four weeks, it can have a negative effect on the latter half (luteal phase) of the menstrual cycle. Your basal body temperature chart can indicate an absence or presence of ovulation and the length of the luteal phase. When your temperature elevation is less than eleven days, it may be due to what physicians call an "inadequate" luteal phase.

Significant enlargement of the ovaries occurs in approximately 5 percent of women a few days after completion of a course of treatment with clomiphene citrate tablets. The longer you're on the drug, the more likely it is. If your ovaries become enlarged or you feel pelvic discomfort, avoid intercourse and physical activity. Your specialist may check you every clomiphene citrate treatment cycle, and also perform an ultrasound examination to look for cysts.

When you do not ovulate even at maximal levels of clomiphene citrate, your specialist may suggest an injection of human chorionic gonadotropin (hCG) at midcycle. This increases LH secretion and may also improve the luteal phase of the cycle. Timing of the hCG injection is important—it usually is given on the seventh day after the last clomiphene citrate tablet. An ultrasound of your ovaries at that time may show a follicle preparing to release an egg. Chances of conception are best on that night and for the following two days.

Most women who have side effects notice them when first taking a 50 mg tablet of the drug, though they are not dose related. Hot flashes—much like those seen in menopausal women—are the most common side effect, occurring in about 10 percent of women. Breast tenderness, bloating, tiredness, headaches, increased acne and hirsutism, depression, nausea, and dryness of scalp hair are less common. Visual symptoms, including blurring or visual spots and flashes, may occur in some women. The length of treatment and an increased dosage of the drug may be also associated with this side effect. Visual symptoms usually disappear within a few days after you stop taking the drug, but can last as long as several weeks. It is usually a good idea to stop treatment if you have this complication.

While there are cautions that patients and doctors should

take seriously, there's good news—very good news—too. Chances are you *can* get pregnant and have a healthy baby. With clomiphene citrate, you can expect the following:

1. The ovulation rate is 80 percent.
2. Approximately 40 percent of the ovulating women become pregnant.
3. The rate of pregnancies per induced ovulatory cycle is 20 to 25 percent.
4. The multiple pregnancy rate is 10 percent—mostly twins, and rarely triplets.

METFORMIN OR CLOMIPHENE CITRATE?

Assuming that the two fertility drugs metformin and clomiphene citrate are more or less equally effective, which is the drug of choice? I recommend metformin because its side effects are potentially less serious than those of clomiphene citrate.

POSSIBLE SIDE EFFECTS

Metformin	Clomiphene Citrate
A third of the women taking it have gastrointestinal symptoms, which usually clear up in three to six weeks.	Breast tenderness, headaches, fatigue, depression.
It crosses the placental barrier to the fetus, although many studies indicate no harm to the fetus.	Increased risk for having twins or triplets.
Lactic acidosis is extremely rare, but can be life-threatening.	Rare but possibly serious ovarian enlargement or ovarian hyperstimulation.
	Rarely, vision changes, severe headaches.
	Increased ovarian testosterone production that may cause further thinning of hair, acne, or body hair growth.

5. The miscarriage rate is not increased.
6. There is no increase in birth defects, and the infant survival rate is normal.
7. If lack of ovulation is the only cause of a woman's infertility, her chance of conceiving over six months is close to the normal rate of 60 to 75 percent.

Some women with PCOS are resistant to this drug, but less so when it's taken in combination with metformin. Women using a combination therapy ovulate and get pregnant more often. In several studies of clomiphene citrate resistant women who were given metformin together with clomiphene citrate, their 10 to 27 percent ovulation rates rose to an average of 80 percent. They also had lower testosterone and insulin levels, a lower BMI, and improved cervical mucus. The addition of metformin to clomiphene citrate probably reduces elevated insulin levels, which are a major factor in the infertility of women with PCOS. This is more likely to occur in very obese women with PCOS and severe insulin resistance.

ACTOS, AVANDIA, AND OTHER DRUGS

Three members of the thiazolidinedione family of drugs have been widely used to treat women with PCOS. In 2000, the FDA banned one of them, troglitazone (Rezulin), because of its potential for liver damage and failure. The other two, pioglitazone (Actos) and rosiglitazone (Avandia), were approved by the FDA in 1999 for the treatment of type 2 diabetes. These drugs operate as well as metformin in achieving ovulation and reducing insulin resistance and elevated testosterone levels. The average dosages of Avandia and Actos in PCOS vary, but often are 4 mg and 30 mg, respectively, taken once daily. Avandia and Actos possibly improve the function of the beta cells of the pancreas that produce insulin. Women may suffer weight gain with these insulin sensitizers, and they reduce insulin resistance even when no weight loss takes place. Before taking these drugs, you need a careful pretreatment evaluation of your liver function. While you are taking them, follow-up liver function studies should be done at three-month intervals for the first year of treatment.

Caution. The problem with these drugs as fertility aids is the open question of how they effect the fetus, since they have not as yet been widely used in women with PCOS. In contrast, most experts agree that metformin has no obvious fetal effects. I do not use these drugs to help women achieve pregnancies. Other strikes against Actos and Avandia are the possibilities of weight gain, headaches, tiredness, and the development of fluid in the legs. A potentially serious complication is that they may cause or worsen heart failure or liver disease. If you do take either drug, be sure to report any rapid increase in weight gain, leg swelling, or shortness of breath to your physician immediately. These drugs are not recommended for women with heart failure and active liver disease.

In otherwise healthy women with PCOS, either of these two drugs may serve as an alternative to those unable to tolerate metformin. Some women who don't respond optimally to metformin alone have more regular menstrual cycles and lower insulin and testosterone levels when they take Actos or Avandia with metformin.

D-Chiro-inositol appears to effectively reduce insulin action in women with PCOS and is virtually free of side effects. There is evidence that it can improve ovulatory function and decrease male hormone levels This option is one to watch for—it's not yet FDA approved or commercially available.

DEXAMETHASONE

An elevated blood level of the male hormone DHEAS in a woman with PCOS is a reliable sign that her adrenal glands (in addition to her ovaries) are secreting increased amounts of male hormones. If your DHEAS level is quite high, and standard treatments for infertility do not work, a small dose of dexamethasone (0.25 mg) can be taken at bedtime with food. This should be used with caution, and only when your endocrinologist and gynecologist agree. It must be stopped as soon as you become pregnant, because there is no uniform consensus on its effect on fetal well-being. This dose can be added to metformin alone, a combination of metformin and clomiphene citrate, or clomiphene citrate alone.

OTHER INFERTILITY OPTIONS

If weight loss through a healthy diet and moderate exercise doesn't work, and if metformin in combination with clomiphene citrate gets no ovarian response, you may need to look at other options. Over the last thirty years, however, only 3 to 4 percent of the infertile women in my practice of nearly 2,000 women with PCOS have needed to resort to in vitro fertilization or similar fertility techniques. The incidence may vary, however, depending on a specialist's type of practice.

A number of techniques and procedures have been developed to solve fertility problems. The following three approaches may be of most interest to women with PCOS.

In vitro fertilization (IVF). A woman's age is important in IVF. The rate of deliveries per egg retrieval is two to three times lower in women over forty than in younger women. As women become older, there is a drop in the number of eggs and they are more vulnerable to problems. Before a woman undergoes IVF, her reproductive endocrinologist usually tests her FSH and estradiol blood levels on day 3 of the menstrual cycle, and again in another cycle if the levels are abnormal, particularly in women over thirty-five. An increase in the FSH level (greater than 20 mIU/ml) and a high estradiol level (over 70 to 100 pg/ml) may indicate a poor likelihood of successful IVF treatment.

In IVF, a number of eggs are surgically removed from a woman's ovaries and fertilized by sperm in vitro (in glass), that is, in a laboratory receptacle. A fertilized egg is implanted in her uterus in the hope that it will develop into a fetus in the natural way. Infants resulting from in vitro fertilization are popularly known as test tube babies. There are more than 1 million test tube babies alive today. The world's first test tube baby, Louise Brown, was born in Britain on July 25, 1978.

Gamete intrafallopian transfer. As with the in vitro fertilization procedure, eggs and sperm are collected from the prospective parents. Instead of being fertilized in vitro, eggs and sperm are inserted by a physician, without surgery, into the woman's uterus. The expectation is that an egg will be fertilized and become implanted in the uterus wall in a natural way.

THE JOURNEY

I hope that throughout your journey you'll remember what I wrote at the start of this chapter—chances are you can get pregnant and have a healthy baby. Sometimes the hardest part is managing expectations and disappointments, so try to keep the big picture in mind and enjoy the sensual pleasures of lovemaking along the way.

[10]

STAYING PREGNANT

If you skipped the last chapter because you're already pregnant, congratulations! The best way to ensure you have a healthy baby—and you can!—is to look after you own body. In my role as a doctor, I have to recommend all the precautions you need to take and warn of the dangers, but don't let these precautions overwhelm you. Don't worry. Motherhood conquers all.

YOUR HEALTHY PREGNANCY

When women with PCOS become pregnant, they need to be more alert than healthy women for possible complications. All pregnant women, particularly those with PCOS, need to be tested for under- or overactive thyroid glands before and after they are pregnant, because they're common and because they can cause powerful hormone imbalances. Some women with PCOS may already have type 2 diabetes, and many are vulnerable to gestational diabetes. In this chapter we'll look at how these two kinds of diabetes can affect pregnancy. High blood pressure is a frequent health problem of women with PCOS and poses additional challenges during pregnancy. It's well known that women with PCOS have a higher miscarriage rate, particularly during the early months of pregnancy, than healthy women. Therefore, we'll also discuss taking metformin as a preventive measure against miscarriages. Finally, we look at the possible effects of a mother's high male hormone level on her female fetus.

Thyroid Function during Pregnancy

The thyroid gland is involved in virtually every body function, and very noticeably in those associated with weight and energy level. Thyroid function lab tests are important for all women, and particularly for pregnant women with PCOS. Once pregnant, you should contact your endocrinologist or obstetrician to schedule thyroid function tests. I perform these tests every three months during a pregnancy.

If an underactive thyroid (hypothyroidism) is not treated during early pregnancy, the fetus may develop neurological abnormalities of the brain. An underactive thyroid may also be responsible for other abnormalities and later cognitive problems. An increase in the blood level of the thyroid-stimulating hormone (TSH) occurs frequently during the first trimester of pregnancy, and you may need to begin taking a thyroid replacement drug.

An overactive thyroid gland (hyperthyroidism) also requires careful follow-up by your endocrinologist, who should prescribe the lowest effective dosage of antithyroid medication. You'll need less of this medication in the third trimester, and lab tests can tell your doctor exactly how much less. Most women with overactive thyroids don't require antithyroid medication at all.

Alert your pediatrician if you are taking thyroid replacement or antithyroid drugs.

TYPE 2 DIABETES

Blood sugar flows freely to the fetus through the placenta, but insulin doesn't. Thus a high maternal blood sugar level triggers a matching insulin response from the developing baby's pancreas, which causes fetal weight gain (macrosomia). Mom's increased blood sugar can also cause anomalies early in pregnancy and even miscarriage. These can all be prevented by tight control of blood sugar levels before and after you conceive. The risk of anomalies increases in the weeks before you give birth, so many medical centers will recommend induced delivery at thirty-eight weeks. With the advent of tight blood sugar control, more and more diabetic women are successfully giving birth to healthy babies.

Many women with PCOS are treated before pregnancy with the insulin-sensitizing medication metformin and other drugs for type 2 diabetes. While there is no evidence that metformin given during pregnancy harms the fetus, it does cross the placenta. Women with PCOS generally have increased insulin resistance during pregnancy, and unfortunately metformin is often not enough to maintain tight blood sugar control in type 2 diabetes. You may need to use insulin therapy, which has been shown to reduce fetal mortality by almost 80 percent in women with type 2 diabetes who do not have PCOS.

While the details of insulin therapy during pregnancy for women with type 2 diabetes are beyond the scope of this book, the following are important goals for pregnant women who have PCOS and either impaired glucose tolerance or type 2 diabetes.

- **Very tight blood sugar control and meticulous management are vital,** especially before conception and during the first seven weeks of pregnancy, when organ development of the fetus takes place.
- **The one-hour postprandial blood glucose level should not exceed 120 mg/dL** during pregnancy. The risk of

weight gain by the fetus increases at levels above 120 mg/dL. Specialists have shown that for women with significant insulin resistance, as in PCOS, a one-hour postprandial blood glucose level not exceeding 110 mg/dL could further reduce potential risks.

- **Your blood glucose level in the fasting state should be below 90 mg/dL.** You should do numerous daily finger sticks with an accurate home monitor to follow your blood glucose levels.

- **Maintain an HbA1c of 5 percent.** Your average blood glucose level over ten to twelve weeks is called the glycosylated hemoglobin A1c (HbA1c). The HbA1c of normal pregnant women drops by 20 percent, to 5 percent or less. With PCOS, the 5 percent range is the target you should aim for. If you find this difficult to achieve, you may need to be referred to a diabetologist or an obstetrician familiar with diabetes during pregnancy.

- **If you have retinal problems due to diabetes, have an ophthalmologist check your eyes** before conception and follow up during pregnancy. Laser photocoagulation may be necessary before becoming pregnant.

Close teamwork of your obstetrician, endocrinologist, and diabetologist is a winning strategy for a healthy pregnancy and to keep the risks to you and the fetus to a minimum.

GESTATIONAL DIABETES

Some women develop high blood sugar levels during pregnancy, a condition known as gestational diabetes. This kind of diabetes typically occurs during the last half of pregnancy, and this is the time when insulin resistance is at its worst. Gestational diabetes usually disappears after pregnancy, but the chances are good that you will develop it again in future pregnancies.

Gestational diabetes occurs in 3 to 5 percent of pregnant women without known PCOS. Most studies show an increased incidence of gestational diabetes in women with PCOS; a few studies put the number at an incredible 40 percent. Estimates vary widely, though, and no large studies have been done to confirm the high end of the range.

It's no surprise that women with PCOS run a greater risk of developing gestational diabetes. In normal women, pregnancy typically increases blood insulin levels anywhere from two and a half to three times. In women with PCOS, that increase comes on top of established insulin resistance, so that the insulin resistance may be increased sevenfold. The insulin-secreting beta cells of the pancreas often simply cannot keep up. Obesity only serves to fuel the insulin resistance fire during pregnancy, and this worsens as pregnancy advances.

The following risk factors for gestational diabetes apply to all pregnant women, with or without PCOS.

- Age greater than thirty
- Insulin resistance prior to pregnancy
- Obesity
- Prior gestational diabetes
- High birth weight of previous child
- Family history of type 2 diabetes
- Smoker
- Native American, African American, Hispanic American, Asian American, or Pacific Islander ethnicity

For some women, gestational diabetes is a first sign of approaching type 2 diabetes. Some specialists claim that one out of every two non-PCOS women develop type 2 diabetes within five years of having had gestational diabetes.

Effective treatment. Since gestational diabetes potentially harms both you and your baby, it's important to start treatment promptly. Treatment may include frequent blood sugar monitoring, insulin injections, special meal plans, and regular physical activity. Your target range for a fasting glucose level should be 60 to 90 mg/L. I always recommend getting the support of a qualified nutritionist and diabetologist or endocrinologist, with experience in treating gestational diabetes.

In a recent study, women with PCOS who took metformin before conception and during pregnancy reduced the rate of gestational diabetes to 7 percent. During pregnancy, metformin reduces insulin resistance, testosterone level, and weight, significantly reducing the complications of gestational diabetes.

For more information on treatment and self-management, see the Web site addresses under Diabetes in the Resources section at the back of the book.

CONTROLLING HIGH BLOOD PRESSURE

High blood pressure (hypertension) is one of the most common medical complications of pregnancy affecting both mother and fetus. Most studies show that pregnant women with PCOS are more likely than normal pregnant women to suffer from high blood pressure, and that those who are obese are at even higher risk. There are four different kinds of high blood pressure diagnoses: chronic hypertension, pre-eclampsia and eclampsia, chronic hypertension with superimposed pre-eclampsia, and gestational hypertension.

Women with chronic hypertension have had an ongoing high blood pressure problem before becoming pregnant. Like many people with high blood pressure, they may not have been aware of it. Many first learn of their condition when searching for help for PCOS, others during a pregnancy checkup.

Pre-eclampsia and eclampsia. Pre-eclampsia consists of a dangerous rise in blood pressure, swelling of the legs, and the

presence of protein in the urine. Some 5 to 8 percent of all pregnant women suffer from this condition, which often begins during week 20 of pregnancy. Delivery may be induced prematurely
when the mother's health is at serious risk. Pre-eclampsia can
cause seizures (eclampsia), kidney and liver damage, internal
bleeding, and poor growth or death of the fetus. Your doctor
should check your blood pressure and urine protein on all prenatal visits. If you do develop pre-eclampsia, you may be prescribed bedrest under managed care until the week 36 of your
pregnancy, when the baby is ready for delivery.

The symptoms of pre-eclampsia and eclampsia include:

- Localized facial swelling of the face or hands
- A weight gain of two or more pounds a week that occurs
  unintentionally
- Headaches
- Nausea, vomiting
- Reduced urine production and the presence of protein in
  the urine
- High blood pressure
- A feeling of being agitated and occasional chest or abdomi-
  nal pains

The risk of pre-eclampsia and eclampsia is three to four
times higher in diabetic women, and this risk is significantly enhanced by poor diabetic control in the first four months of pregnancy. Risk factors for pre-eclampsia include the following—the
first three put women with PCOS at particular risk.

- High blood pressure before pregnancy
- Type 2 diabetes before pregnancy
- African-American women
- Obesity before pregnancy
- Twins or triplets

- Pregnancy after age forty
- Pregnancy before age twenty
- Kidney disease, rheumatoid arthritis, lupus, scleroderma

If you have any of these risk factors, talk to your doctor—preferably before you become pregnant. Lowering your high blood pressure is probably the most important preventive step you can take.

Becoming pregnant late in life and having twins or triplets, after help from a fertility clinic, are a combination of risk factors responsible for increasing numbers of pre-eclampsia cases.

Chronic hypertension with superimposed pre-eclampsia. This third type of high blood pressure in pregnant women is more likely to develop when high blood pressure occurs early in pregnancy and worsens as it progresses. Unfortunately, this condition may lead to the placenta separating from the lining of the uterus before the usual time, causing pain, bleeding, and all too often miscarriage, though caesarean delivery can sometimes save the baby.

Gestational hypertension. In this condition, high blood pressure develops about halfway through pregnancy, but no proteins are excreted in the urine. Blood pressure usually returns to normal two to three months after delivery. Women with PCOS have a 12 percent incidence rate of pregnancy-induced hypertension compared with a 1.3 percent rate for normal women.

Treatment. You can lower your high blood pressure by losing 10 percent of your body weight, avoiding salt, and exercising regularly. Keep in mind that most doctors advise against taking ACE inhibitors and most other drugs for high blood pressure while you are pregnant.

LOSING A PREGNANCY

Sadly, women with PCOS have three times the normal risk for early miscarriage, which is 10 to 15 percent in normal women. Of women who repeatedly miscarry in the first trimester, up to four out of five have been reported to have PCOS. There is hope for these women, though, in the form of the insulin-sensitizing medication metformin.

Metformin is recognized by the FDA as a Category B drug, which means that it has caused no fetal abnormalities in animal studies. Treatment with metformin often enables women with PCOS infertility to conceive, as we discussed in the previous chapter, and continued use during the first trimester may significantly reduce the chance of an early miscarriage. In one study, women with PCOS who continued metformin for the first trimester had a normal miscarriage rate (8.8 percent), while similar women who did not take metformin had a 42 percent miscarriage rate.

Metformin decreases high insulin levels, high male hormone levels, and possibly obesity. It reduces blood clotting and increases the levels of two protective proteins in the uterus lining.

Women with PCOS who have had three or more miscarriages have given birth after treatment with metformin for the first three months of pregnancy, and occasionally throughout pregnancy. Although metformin is not known to cause any fetal or birth defects, doctors must still hesitate to recommend this extended usage until more long-range studies show that it's safe.

I recommend that a woman with PCOS who has not been pregnant before discontinue metformin when she conceives. If she has already had one or more miscarriages, she should have the option of continuing metformin for the first trimester. However, a large randomized clinical trial of women is necessary to establish that this is the best option for these women.

SAVING YOUR SKIN AND HAIR FROM PCOS

In this chapter, we look at treatments for the skin and hair symptoms that my patients understandably find so troubling: acne, excess facial and body hair, and thinning scalp hair. We also talk about how to control your symptoms while you are waiting for medications to take effect.

Taking metformin to reverse infertility, as we discussed in chapter 9, lowers your insulin resistance and male hormone levels, and can be helpful for skin and hair problems, too. If you're trying to get pregnant you'll need to steer clear of some of the treatments I recommend in this chapter—oral contraceptives, for starters. You should also not use drugs to lower the level of male hormones (antiandrogen drugs) for four to six months before you take a fertility drug, because of the damage they can cause to a growing fetus.

SEE YOUR WAY CLEAR

As distressing as it is for many women with PCOS, acne is usually not difficult to treat. When it's mild to moderate, a fair number of women respond to oral contraceptives, but that's not the end of your treatment options.

ORAL CONTRACEPTIVES

Oral contraceptives are effective weapons against acne in part because they reduce male hormones secretions from your ovaries. Individual women respond differently to different contraceptives, so don't abandon hope if the first one your doctor prescribes doesn't work or even worsens the problem. Just move on to the next.

Sometimes switching from one oral contraceptive to another is all that is needed to improve your skin. An oral contraceptive containing 0.03 mg ethinyl estradiol (a synthetic estrogen) and 3.0 mg of the antiandrogenic progestin drospirenone (brand name Yasmin) has been effective in the treatment of cystic acne. Many women who use Yasmin for moderate or severe acne also need to take an antiandrogen, because one Yasmin tablet contains a relatively small dose of the ingredient that fights acne.

Before you start oral contraceptive therapy:

- **Make sure you are not already pregnant.**
- **Consider your medical history.** Severe varicose veins, high blood pressure, or severe migraines may mean oral contraceptives are a bad choice for you. Oral contraceptives increase the risk of phlebitis in overweight women. Also, while there is no clear evidence that women who take oral contraceptives are at higher risk of breast cancer, it may be *slightly* higher in women with a mother or sibling with breast cancer.

- **Be prepared to quit smoking.** Oral contraceptives and cigarettes are a bad combination. The clotting effect of smoking enhances the risk of heart attack, stroke, phlebitis, and the possible passage of a blood clot from the legs to the lungs.
- **Consider other side effects.** Oral contraceptives may promote mild weight gain, and in many women some degree of mood changes. Sometimes, switching to another oral contraceptive may be helpful. Side effects and mood changes due to contraceptives vary from person to person.

On the plus side, oral contraceptives:

- **Reduce the incidence of ovarian and uterine cancers.** This is important for women with PCOS, who have a higher incidence of uterine cancer than other women.
- **Reduce the levels of testosterone and free testosterone** by suppressing the hypothalamus and pituitary stimulation of ovarian hormone secretion.
- **Reduce the incidence of ovarian and uterine cancers.**

If You Have Acne . . .

Everyone these days seems to be an expert on skin care—women's magazines, books, and Web sites all offer advice on keeping your skin young and fresh looking. Yet in spite of it all, many women still harbor misconceptions about how to effectively fight acne. Part of your daily routine may actually be aggravating the problem. Here are a few things to avoid:

1. Excessive washing and scrubbing may worsen acne. It certainly won't make blackheads go away.
2. Squeezing pimples doesn't help acne and may even cause permanent scarring. Leave them be!
3. Sunscreens can be bad for acne. Look for products labeled *noncomedogenic,* which means that they are unlikely to cause whiteheads or blackheads.

SPIRONOLACTONE (ALDACTONE)

For moderate to severe acne, the most commonly used antiandrogen in the United States is spironolactone (Aldactone). It is taken twice a day, often in 50 to 75 mg doses at mealtimes, for a total daily dose of 100 to 150 mg. Most women on this dosage notice improvement in cystic acne three to four months after they start taking the drug.

While spironolactone is an effective drug for severe acne, its side effects can make its benefits hard earned. Before you decided to take it, consider the following:

- **Periodic blood testing required.** Spironolactone has been used as a diuretic for about fifty years. It may cause increased salt excretion by blocking the effect of an adrenal hormone called aldosterone and it may cause potassium retention. If you decide to use this drug, you'll need periodic blood tests for electrolytes, including potassium. In rare instances, the blood potassium level may rise and cause muscle cramps and discomfort. For that reason, it is best to avoid antihypertensive drugs such as angiotensin-converting enzyme (ACE) inhibitor—for example, enalapril (brand name Vasotec)—when you're taking spironolactone. You can still eat foods containing potassium because a normal intake of the mineral does not contribute to a rise in the blood level of potassium.
- **Stay hydrated.** Make sure you do not become dehydrated or low in salt in hot weather or during strenuous exercise. I recommend eating saltine crackers, a small sour pickle, or any other salty snack before exercise. Drinking excessive amounts of water without salt can dilute the level of sodium in your body and can lead to dizziness and in rare cases water intoxication.
- **Spironolactone may make you dizzy** when you bend over rapidly or stand quickly, especially if you have a tendency to

low blood pressure. If this happens, have your physician check your blood pressure while sitting and then quickly standing up. A significant drop in blood pressure may indicate the need for either a reduced dosage of spironolactone or more salt in your diet.

- **Use with an oral contraceptive,** that is, unless an oral contraceptive is a bad choice for you because of your medical history. If you don't use birth control and then become pregnant, you risk damaging the growing fetus. About half the women who take spironolactone without an oral contraceptive have two menstrual cycles a month. This is especially common among women who take at least two 50 mg doses a day or more.

- **Some women complain of occasional headaches, mood changes, drowsiness, and breast tenderness.** Some women report that their breasts become enlarged. No increased risk of breast cancer, however, has been documented.

- **Frequently, a reduced sex drive occurs.** A lower sex drive often accompanies lower blood testosterone levels, particularly when spironolactone is used with an oral contraceptive.

- **Increased urinary frequency** is an annoying symptom that can be lessened by drinking water at times that do not interfere with getting the sleep you need.

SKIN ABSCESS THERAPY

About 3 to 4 percent of women with PCOS develop small abscesses caused by blocked sweat glands under the skin. They often require the use of antibiotics. Boils under the arms, if large and recurrent, may have to be drained and removed. If left untreated, this constant source of infection may lead to immunological responses, including arthritis and a condition called amyloidosis.

- **Before starting spironolactone treatment, be sure you are not pregnant and will not wish to be for six months after treatment.** For the few women who use spironolactone without oral contraceptives, this is mandatory.

ACCUTANE AND BENZACLIN

In instances of severe acne, dermatologists often recommend isotretinoin (Accutane), but its side effects are significant, and several treatments of four to six months are necessary. Before using Accutane, be sure you are not pregnant, and don't become pregnant while using it. The side effects include dry lips and skin, and about one woman in ten has some shedding of scalp hair. Less common side effects include depression, feelings of aggression, skeletal and muscle discomfort, and changes and difficulties in vision due mostly to dry eyes.

To reduce the hundreds of miscarriages, birth defects, and abortions associated with Accutane each year, an FDA regulation requires that, as of December 31, 2005, patients taking Accutane and doctors prescribing it must register with manufacturers of the drug and promise to comply with instructions for its use.

The prescription drug Benzaclin topical gel is a popular ini-

TRIPLE THERAPY

Women with high insulin levels and irregular periods who are distressed by severe acne, excess facial and body hair, or loss of scalp hair and who do *not* want to conceive have the option of triple therapy. This consists of a combination of metformin, an oral contraceptive, and spironolactone or another antiandrogen. Triple therapy is very effective for severe skin and hair symptoms in insulin resistant women with PCOS, regardless of their weight. My patients have used triple therapy successfully, but this option means my patient and I need to be extra vigilant about monitoring side effects.

tial treatment for acne. From 15 to 20 percent of the women who use it develop dry skin.

UNWANTED HAIR

As a first step you can try oral contraceptives on their own to control excessive growth of facial and body hair, but chances are you'll need some kind of combination therapy. Only 10 percent or less of women respond well, that is, notice a a significant reduction in hair growth. A combination of oral contraceptives and spironolactone (or other antiandrogen drug) is much more effective. For women with moderate to severe hirsutism, a total daily divided dosage not exceeding 200 mg of spironolactone usually brings things under control, though you may not notice significant improvement (e.g., you only need one electrolysis session a month instead of two) until you've been taking the drugs for four to six months. The hair that does return is also finer and lighter in color. Length of treatment varies, depending on how well you respond and whether you wish to conceive. If you do decide you want to get pregnant, stop taking spironolactone at least six months before your first attempt to conceive.

Women with severe hirsutism who do not respond to other forms of treatment have responded to an injection of gonadotropin-releasing hormone (GnRH) agonist combined with an oral contraceptive. I don't recommend injections alone because of the risk of significant bone loss.

OTHER ANTIANDROGENS

Other antiandrogens include 5a-reductase inhibitors and flutamide. Outside the United States, Diane (a combination of an estrogen and the antiandrogen-progestin cyproterone acetate) is reported to be equal and sometimes superior to the combination of an oral contraceptive and spironolactone. Cyproterone acetate, however, has not been approved by the FDA for use in the United States. Insulin-sensitizing agents, such as metformin, may cause some improvement in hirsutism, but in my experience it takes at least nine to twelve months for any visible improvement.

5a-reductase inhibitors. These include finasteride (Proscar) and dutasteride (Avodart), which work by suppressing 5 alpha-reductase, the enzyme that converts testosterone to its active form, DHT, at the site of hair growth. While the drugs have been judged safe to use for other purposes, they have *not* been approved by the FDA for this use in women. In other words, the studies required for approval have not been conducted, though a few reports claim that 5a-reductase inhibitors can be helpful in treating hirsutism and scalp hair loss. The dosage for effective treatment with finasteride was between 2.5 and 7.5 mg daily, while that of dutasteride is 0.5 mg daily. They are mostly used when a treatment with a combination of an oral contraceptive and spironolactone fail. Women with liver problems or abnormal liver chemistries (lab results) should not use 5a-reductase inhibitors, nor should women of reproductive age without the protection of contraceptives, because of the very serious risk of potential of birth defects of fetal male genitalia. Women I have treated with 5a-reductase inhibitors have had few side effects, and the inhibitors work well in controlling scalp hair loss. As of this writing, no large-scale study of their use and effectiveness in women with PCOS has been published. Of the two drugs, it appears to me that dutasteride may be more effective for severe hirsutism and scalp hair loss than finasteride. I have prescribed a combination of dutasteride, spironolactone, and oral contraceptives only when a woman has been very seriously affected by these symptoms.

Flutamide (Eulexin). It is considered by many endocrinologists to be the best antiandrogen available. It works by blocking the binding of testosterone to its receptors, while also affecting the hypothalamus and pituitary. The results are more regular menstrual cycles. The dosage varies, but a low dose of a 125 mg capsule twice a day is usually effective for severe skin or hair symptoms due to PCOS, though some women may need a higher dose—250 mg twice a day. Anyone with a history of liver disease or chemical liver function abnormalities should not take this drug. Like spironolactone, it has not been approved by the FDA for the treatment of hirsutism.

Unfortunately, diarrhea is a frequent side effect. Flutamide, because it can potentially damage your liver, requires careful supervision by the doctor who prescribes it for you. You should report any darkening of your urine, flu-like symptoms, or body itch to your doctor and immediately stop taking the drug. If you take this drug you'll need regular liver function lab tests, though you may well notice something is not right before a lab test confirms it. I have prescribed flutamide reluctantly for a very small group of patients, because nothing else has been effective in treating their hair loss. The patients avoided becoming pregnant and, with full understanding, balanced its benefits against its risk of the rare but serious side effect of liver failure.

VANIQA

A cream made of 13.9 percent eflornithine hydrochloride (Vaniqa) has been approved by the FDA for the treatment of unwanted facial hair. You apply Vaniqa to your chin and lower portions of your face twice a day. This cream is meant to be used on your face, and on your face only. It blocks an enzyme that permits hair follicles to develop, but has no depilatory effect—that is, it won't dissolve or get rid of the hair you already have. Generally women start to notice results about three months after they start using the cream. Vaniqa works for most women, and its main side effect is a burning sensation or rash on the skin being treated.

TRIED AND TRUE MEANS

Most women take measures to remove unwanted facial and body hair long before they ask me for help. And they often continue doing so for some time after. It can be weeks or even months before you see visible improvement from drug therapy. The following are some of the mechanical hair removal options readily available.

Shaving. It's a myth that shaving makes hair grow thicker and faster. Warm water, plenty of soap lather, and a sharp blade produce the best results. Electric razors eliminate nicks, but the shave is not as close and electric razors often causes skin irritation or a rash until your skin becomes accustomed to it.

Bleaching. Facial or body hairs bleached to match your skin color become almost invisible—a nice solution if your skin doesn't react to the bleach.

Pumice. You can remove fine hair with a pumice stone. I hope I don't need to tell you not to rub too hard or you will irritate your skin. Wash the area afterward and apply a moisturizer.

Plucking. Because it is slow and painful, plucking with tweezers is usually only for facial hair. Plucking can also irritate or infect hair follicles. The hair-free period following plucking with tweezers is much longer than that after shaving.

Depilatories. Over-the-counter depilatories are available as creams, lotions, gels, roll-ons, and sprays. You leave a depilatory on your skin for a few minutes (check individual product labels for instructions) and then wipe it off, removing unwanted hair with it. Follow the instructions carefully. Depilatories suitable for your body or legs may not be so for your face. They can cause skin irritation and should not be used on skin cuts or rashes.

Waxing. Salons and spas offer this hair removal treatment, though you can do it yourself at home. You apply melted wax on your skin, let it cool, then pull it off, removing embedded hairs with it. As in plucking with tweezers, irritated or infected follicles can result.

Electrolysis. An electrologist inserts a probe at each hair root and kills the hair follicle with a small electrical charge. Electrologists may use one of three methods: (1) direct-current electrolysis; (2) alternating-current thermolysis; or (3) a blend of both. If this sounds like a risky procedure, you're not far off: In the hands of anyone but a skilled professional, it is. Skin scars, electric shock, and infections can result if it not done properly. It is worthwhile to check the qualifications of anyone who is treating you with electrolysis and determine if she or he is a member of the major professional electrology group, such as the American Electrology Association (AEA). Look into whether your state has a licensing procedure for electrologists. The AEA has voluntary tests and continuing education for professionals. Ask him or her directly about qualifications, experience, and references and rely on your own observations as to whether the person is responsible and clean, has sterile instruments, wears surgical gloves, and so forth. Professionals should use sterilized, single-use disposable needles and practice other precautions, including hand washing and disposable gloves for each treatment.

Hair does not grow back after successful electrolysis, though hair roots not exactly under the hair follicle openings cannot be successfully treated with electrolysis (at least initially). So while it's a slow and expensive process, it's worthwhile for many women.

Only a small area of skin is treated on each visit. The number of treatments will vary with hair growth cycles, the quantity and structure of hair being removed, hormonal function, and certain medications. Often some scabbing occurs—a normal and healthy part of the healing process. If you become pregnant, discuss with your physician whether you should continue the use of electrolysis. I recommend that my patients stop.

Home kits for electrolysis are available, but their results do not compare with those achievable by a skilled professional.

Laser hair removal. The FDA has approved laser hair removal, but not claims that the hair removal is "permanent." That said, laser treatment for a year and a half may produce a 90 percent reduction in hair growth. Initially, for each skin area, you have to have three to five treatments about a month apart. To achieve optimal results, you may need up to eight treatments or more for each skin area. Although laser therapy is more expensive than electrolysis, the skin area treated on each visit is larger and treatment is less time-consuming.

Lasers work on actively growing hair. At any given time, up to a third of the hair follicles in a given area may be dormant and thus unaffected by the treatment. Do not pluck or wax a skin area before laser treatment, because this removes hairs from follicles; it is okay to shave. Lasers work best on women with light skin. It can be helpful to dye blond hairs dark and to wait for deep tans to fade before you have a treatment.

Laser hair removal doesn't hurt. Some women describe it as akin to having a rubber band snapped against your skin. A topical anesthetic cream can be given in advance if you're highly sensitive. The area is cleaned and shaved prior to laser treatment. The laser energy passes through the skin and is absorbed by the pigment in the hair follicle. The skin area treated may become slightly reddened or irritated for a day or so. Women with dark skin or a deep tan may have some temporary lightening of skin color. For at least a week before each treatment, avoid medications that make your skin more sensitive to light (tetracycline, St. John's wort) or lasers (skin care products such as Retin A, Renova cream, and other glycolic or alpha-hydroxy acid preparations). Sun screens are recommended for any area that is to be treated.

NIPPLE DISCHARGE THERAPY

Perhaps 7 percent of women with PCOS complain of nipple discharge (galactorrhea), usually in association with infrequent menstrual cycles and hirsutism. The nipple discharge is usually caused by an elevated prolactin blood level, which is due to overactivity of prolactin-secreting pituitary cells (lactotropes) and the presence of pituitary microadenoma that may or may not be found on MRI testing. Some drugs may cause a milky white discharge from the breasts as well. These include a variety of psychotropic drugs, which may increase the prolactin level to some extent. Thorazine, Compazine, and, to a lesser extent, Prozac and verapamil may increase the prolactin blood level. Stopping the drugs, when possible, will cause the nipple discharge to lessen or disappear.

Bromocriptine (Parlodel) is the best treatment. Bromocriptine lowers the prolactin blood level, improves menstrual function, and lightens mood disturbances. After two to three months of treatment, its effectiveness should be assessed. Bromocriptine can be taken at meals in combination with ovulation-promoting medications. Nipple discharge does not always occur when a woman's prolactin blood level is high. Normal levels of prolactin may occur in association with a milky breast discharge. If a woman is unable to tolerate the initial nausea and light-headedness of bromocriptine, she may tolerate dostinex (Cabergoline) better.

HAIR PATROL

Thinning scalp hair (alopecia) is a traumatic event for any woman. As I mentioned in chapter 1, your scalp becomes visible through your hair after about 20 percent of your scalp hair has been lost. The incidence of alopecia in PCOS varies from 40 to 67 percent. It's most visible toward the front and top of the head.

Before you hold PCOS responsible, you and your doctor should consider other possible causes. For example, vegetarians who have not eaten any red meat for a relatively long period may have a reduced zinc blood level and consequent hair loss. Genetic, local, age-related, nutritional, chronic diseases, and hormonal factors have to be taken into account. Androgen excess diseases, thyroid diseases (including hypo- and hyperthyroidism), and anemias have to be excluded. Hair loss can be due to a protein deficiency, or deficiencies in folic acid, B-12, or other B-complex vitamins caused by a poor diet or an associated medical condition. An iron deficiency, due to lack of red meat in the diet or heavy menstrual bleeding, may also cause hair loss.

DRUGS THAT CAN CAUSE OR WORSEN HAIR LOSS

- Corticosteroids (cortisone-like drugs) taken orally, and sometimes the chronic use of topical cortisone preparations for skin conditions
- Lithium carbonate
- Levodopa
- Propranolol or atenolol (brand names Inderal and Tenormin)
- Anti-neoplastic agents
- Cyclosporine
- Propylthioracil (PTU) and another antithyroid drug, methimazole (brand name Tapazole)
- Cimetidine (brand name Tagamet)
- Danazol (used in the treatment of endometriosis)
- Accutane

Of all the skin and hair problems women with PCOS struggle with, scalp hair loss is probably the most difficult to treat. There are drugs that can help reduce loss—specifically a daily dose of spironolactone (no more than 200 mg) and an oral contraceptive.

When scalp hair loss is caused by elevated male hormone levels, it's difficult to regrow. Sometimes fine hair comes back, but unfortunately that's uncommon. The best thing you can to is catch it early and get treatment to prevent further loss as soon as possible.

Other treatments for women with PCOS and scalp hair loss involve combining an oral contraceptive with finasteride (Proscar) or dutasteride (Avodart), to which spironolactone may sometimes be added.

Outside the United States, women with alopecia, hirsutism, or acne can use cyproterone acetate, which has not been approved by the FDA, though it's been used elsewhere for more than thirty years. The FDA may have concerns regarding an increased incidence of phlebitis and thrombotic tendencies and, rarely, adrenal insufficiency. It is combined with ethinyl estradiol in different drugs (Dianette, Diane-35) for women with elevated male hormone levels and alopecia. Diane-35 has resulted in modest improvements in more than half of thirty patients with scalp hair loss that I have followed up. Most of these women went to Canada, where I referred them to an endocrinologist who uses this drug. Experts disagree on the comparative anti-androgenic effects of cyproterone acetate and spironolactone. Generally they seem about equally effective, with cyproterone acetate being minimally more effective in the treatment of scalp hair loss in women with elevated male hormone levels.

The use of minoxidil (brand name Rogaine) in the treatment of alopecia is modestly useful. It must be used daily, however. Take great care with this product—you don't want any of the solution to drip onto your face. Remember, it promotes hair growth!

Keep in mind that heredity often plays a major role in determining the degree of hair loss and its response to treatment. Normal daily scalp hair loss is between 100 and 150 hairs, and cutting back on the number of times you wash your hair a week won't affect your hair loss problems.

Some women lose hair seasonally—that is, they shed more hair in the spring and fall months. Also, a woman starts losing some scalp hair as she approaches menopause. This onset of hair loss is visible in many women after the age of forty.

I recommend the following for the care of thinning scalp hair:

- Avoid tugging your hair or anything that causes tugging, such as a headband, braids, or ponytail.
- Don't play with your hair or curls.
- Don't use hot or fairly warm blow dryers.
- Eat a balanced diet.

THE EMOTIONAL IMPACT OF PCOS

Dealing with the most visible signs of PCOS is no walk in the park. In fact, for some, the social consequences of excessive hair growth, acne, and thinning scalp hair are traumatic—there's just no other word for it, as studies I'll talk about in the following pages show. Many also have to face the added burden of being overweight or obese and the possibility of long-term health risks that come with it. So it's no surprise that many of my patients are anxious, stressed-out, and frustrated.

In early adolescence, girls with PCOS—like many other girls that age—are dissatisfied with the way they look. They hate being different from their friends who have a relatively clear complexion and normal body weight. And the feeling that they don't fit in shapes many aspects of their life. They may become obsessed with their body image and feel less than feminine.

In our culture, girls learn early to tie self-esteem to certain body shapes (the thinner the better!) and flawless skin, and that idea is only reinforced by the media. Ads for everything from soap to bikinis can be painful reminders for young women, especially those with PCOS, that they fall short of the mark. The fictional fairyland of skinny, toned, and smooth-skinned beauties is real to young girls, and this makes it that much harder for them to cope with their physical symptoms.

In this environment, it can be difficult for them to understand what is happening to them. If other family members are overweight, they may have learned that genes play a significant role in body shape and they may even start blaming their parents for their weight problems.

Poor self-esteem and dissatisfaction with body image can lead to varying degrees of depression in girls, and in those with PCOS in particular. Some girls cope by exercising rigid control over what they can—namely, what they eat. When taken to extremes, they develop a variety of eating disorders that can have serious medical consequences. Quite thin, clinically hirsute women with eating disorders such as anorexia nervosa or bulimia make up 2 to 3 percent of my PCOS patients. They have the clinical features of PCOS, including elevated male hormone blood levels and polycystic ovaries visible on ultrasound. They're typically fat-phobic and are obsessive about avoiding dietary fats. Their chronic eating disorders often persist until the late twenties and early thirties.

Since PCOS often becomes evident at the same age girls become interested in attracting romantic partners, the cosmetic and psychosexual effects of the syndrome usually cause profound emotional distress.

STUDIES SHOW YOU'RE NOT ALONE

In a British study of heterosexual women in a PCOS self-help group, G. Kitzinger and J. Wilmott found that PCOS had a major impact in the daily life of most of the thirty participants who volunteered to be the subjects of in-depth interviews. Many spoke about the frustration and anger resulting from delay in diagnosis, the lack of information they received from health professionals, and the frustration of trying to get doctors to take their symptoms seriously. Many researched their symptoms and strongly suspected PCOS as a probable cause long before seeing a series of physicians. They were assertive in asking for specific treatments, and this sometimes led to problems in doctor-patient relationships.

They repeatedly referred to themselves as "freaks" and felt they failed to conform to "normal" womanhood or "femininity." Their most distressing symptoms were excessive facial and body hair, menstrual irregularity, and infertility. Many were reassured through group meetings that others with PCOS actually looked quite normal and feminine, beyond a few facial hairs. The idea that they had increased levels of male hormones conjured up many negative feelings and having to remove facial hair was a constant reminder of their supposed lack of femininity. Some went to great lengths to hide their facial hair from husbands or close friends.

In the same study, erratic periods or sometimes heavy and frequent menstrual bleeding were also distressing symptoms. Some said it was hard to feel like a woman with only a few periods a year. Others said that the menstrual cycle is a fundamental part of being a woman, and not having a period regularly made them feel "odd" or "like a child." They often considered the use of birth control pills as "artificial" and offering a "fake" sense of femininity.

My patients often echo these feelings, and believe pills are unhealthy and unfeminine. Infertility promoted powerful, crushing feelings of failure. Women in the study were, to some extent, reassured that even "normal" women at times have difficulty conceiving. Still, they carried a sense of shame linked to their trouble conceiving, and fertility treatments were generally kept secret even from close friends and family.

A review of the effects of PCOS on health-related quality of life was published by S. Coffey and H. Mason in 2003. Since the experience of life and therefore illness is subjective, the measurement of how the illness affects you and the benefits to you of treatment are vital in the understanding of PCOS. During psychological testing, women with PCOS had higher levels of the adrenal stress hormone cortisol compared with those in a control group, indicating an increased incidence of depression, psychosexual problems, and anxiety. Hirsutism and acne can affect quality of life in the same way severe chronic illnesses can. (When women with PCOS have type 2 diabetes, diabetic complications affect their quality of life immensely.) On the other hand, any improvements in skin and hair symptoms resulted in dramatic improvements in quality of life.

In a German survey published in 2003 by Dr. Onno Janssen and others, fifty women with PCOS and control subjects were interviewed. Hirsutism, obesity, and infertility had significant psychological disturbances, which included the following:

- Interpersonal sensitivity
- Depression
- Obsessive-compulsive behavior
- Frustration and anxiety
- Aggression
- Vitality
- Poor social function
- Less satisfaction with sex life and a negative feeling of sexual self-worth
- Feeling less attractive

In my experience, weight loss, reduced male hormone levels, and improved PCOS symptoms profoundly improve emotional well-being.

DEPRESSION

Most cases of depression go both undiagnosed and untreated, perhaps because people hide their depression well. They hold down jobs, but when home alone, they can feel so depressed, they are almost incapacitated. They take pleasure in nothing, have little appetite, and often sleep poorly. They don't go out socially and may sit in front of the TV all evening without really watching anything. A few of them sleep the time away. The next morning, they put on a cheerful face for another day at work. For some, this feeling of depression passes after some weeks or months. Others need professional help, and the sooner the better.

In all of our lives, things happen that make us feel sad, such as the death of a loved one, divorce, or job loss. Sadness is an understandable reaction to such events. Although your sadness may be intense, you carry on with your life. As time passes, your feelings lighten.

When your sadness doesn't lift with time and starts to interfere with your work and social relationships, you have developed what psychiatrists call a mood disorder. Depression at this level requires professional care.

About one in ten Americans become depressed at some time each year, affecting one out of five families. Nearly two-thirds of depressed people don't realize it. Among those who do know, some are ashamed, seeing depression as personal weakness or a character flaw. Relatively few receive adequate treatment. You needn't be one of them!

NINA AND ANGELA

When Nina and Angela were laid off, friends couldn't help noticing the difference in the way each handled the situation. They had worked for the same company and knew each other well through belonging to the same PCOS support group. Their husbands got along, their kids went to the same school district—they'd even vacationed together.

Financially the layoffs hit both families hard. After several months of searching for a job that would replace her lost income, Nina took a municipal job at a significant pay cut. The family watched the purse strings more closely but continued to enjoy their lives.

Angela had no more success than Nina in finding a good job, but she didn't settle for a step down in pay. After some months, she began sleeping most of the day, paying little attention to her children or house. She sometimes went shopping for hours, but never bought anything. She began gaining weight through compulsive eating, and her PCOS symptoms worsened.

Nina persuaded her friend to see a psychiatrist, in spite of her fears that family and friends might think she was "going crazy." Angela was diagnosed with major depression and subsequently recovered with the help of antidepressants. Her psychiatrist suggested that she might have been already suffering from PCOS-related depression before the layoffs—the event had simply triggered major depression.

With effective treatment, Angela was soon surprised at how much better she felt.

Are More Women Than Men Depressed?

In a word, probably. Twice as many women as men are diagnosed with depression, though equal numbers of very young boys and girls become depressed; it's in adolescence that more girls than boys become depressed. This greater likelihood of depression continues through women's lives into old age. Some women may respond to stress differently than men. Others may have more stress. Women's roles in both workplace and home can involve more worries and conflicts.

On the other hand, women may be diagnosed more frequently because of their greater willingness to see a doctor. They are also more willing than men to acknowledge their feelings. Men may repress feelings of depression or mask them with alcohol or drug abuse. Where alcohol and drugs are not available, men and women are diagnosed with depression with more or less the same frequency.

Hormonal changes during menstrual cycles may be associated with depression in some women. The hormonal changes of pregnancy and childbirth can also precipitate mood changes. Women who become depressed at menopause, however, typically have had previous episodes of depression.

Therefore, although we know that twice as many women as men are diagnosed with depression, we cannot be sure that more women than men suffer from the condition.

Red Flags

There are no test strips or lab tests to show that you have major depression. Instead, doctors rely on the presence of four kinds of symptoms to make a diagnosis. These are:

- Mood
- Behavior
- Thinking patterns
- Physical symptoms

These symptoms vary with personality and age. For example, the most noticeable symptom is often a change in behavior in the young, a persistent bad mood in the middle-aged, and physical symptoms in the elderly. Some people feel worse in the early morning and better later in the day. Women may be more depressed before the onset of menstruation.

When diagnosing depression, doctors look for at least five of the nine following symptoms. A depressed mood must be predominant, last for at least two weeks, and be severe enough to interfere with daily activities.

Depressed mood. This low mood can be so strong that you may not remember what it was like to feel otherwise. You may resent anyone who offers advice or help, or drive people away, socially isolating yourself as your mood worsens.

Sleep disturbance. Four out of five people with major depression have sleep problems. Some find it hard to fall asleep, while others wake during the night and remain awake. A few escape into long periods of sleep.

Loss of interest. You lose interest in the small things that previously added fun to your life. Family and friends notice your loss of interest and pleasure in them. You also lose interest in the pleasures of sex. A lowered sex drive is frequently a warning of oncoming depression.

Feelings of guilt and hopelessness. Your guilt is excessive, inappropriate, and sometimes even delusional. Guilt is often accompanied by excessive feelings of hopelessness, helplessness, or worthlessness.

Fatigue. You feel tired much of the time and don't have enough energy to accomplish everyday things you once did without thinking much about. Your work declines, the laundry piles up, and much gets postponed.

Concentration difficulties. You have difficulty concentrating, thinking logically, or making decisions. You may suffer from some memory loss. Depression can affect your judgment, sometimes making you wonder why you did something that you normally would not do.

Appetite decrease or increase. You may lose your appetite, hardly notice food anymore, or even be nauseated by the thought of it. Your loss of appetite may cause you to lose more than 5 percent loss of your body weight in a month. Some depressed people gain weight through increased appetite and sugar cravings. This is more likely to occur in hormonal disturbances such as PCOS, Cushing's syndrome, and thyroid disorders.

Slow or agitated movement. Depression can slow you down. You may speak more slowly and take more time to respond. You may walk around with slumped shoulders and eyes on the ground, avoiding eye contact. Older people are more likely to develop agitated movements. They may not be able to sit still, so they pace, wringing their hands and gesturing nervously.

Suicidal thinking. If you're feeling so low that suicide seems like a solution, tell your family and friends as soon as possible and seek professional help, whether or not you've actually made plans about how you would do it.

Effective Help

If you are feeling depressed, don't hunker down and hope the feeling will pass. Perhaps it won't. You can be helped. If you think you can't, that is your depressed self thinking, not the real you. If you have major depression, you need professional help, so ask your family doctor for a referral—he or she will keep the referral confidential, if you request that. You need not acknowledge visits to a psychiatrist as *psychiatric treatment* on future legal or employment records.

Seeing a psychiatrist today does not involve long hours on a couch recalling incidents from childhood. Chances are, once a psychiatrist diagnoses you with major depression, his or her immediate task will be to get you feeling better as soon as possible. Finding the cause of your depression is much less important than restoring your sense of well-being. The psychiatrist might prescribe antidepressants. Only after you have begun to respond positively will treatment proceed further. As a woman with

PCOS, you need to help the psychiatrist at the outset by suggesting that your symptoms are a cause, if they are, of your depression.

Why a psychiatrist? Aren't there other qualified professionals, and remedies other than antidepressants? Yes, indeed, there may be other effective alternatives. However, if you are already depressed, you need rapid treatment to help you out of it. In my experience, psychiatrists and antidepressants have proved themselves as a reliable rescue means in an emergency.

ANXIETY

Women with skin and hair problems caused by PCOS are likely to have strong feelings of anxiety, and to be even more aware of them than feelings of depression. Such anxiety is natural and does not amount to an emotional disorder. Feeling anxious in this way is equivalent to feeling sad over a loss. Both are appropriate emotions, until they become overwhelming and interfere with daily activities.

People with anxiety strong enough to qualify as an emotional disorder often feel apprehension or fear about a danger they have not yet perceived—they have a feeling something *could* happen. Shortness of breath, a rapid heartbeat, trembling, and sweating are among the physical symptoms of anxiety.

Many depressed people also suffer from anxiety. Women with PCOS frequently experience some combination of the two. When a woman's depression is lifted by an antidepressant, her anxiety tends to disappear also. If her anxiety persists or if she suffers from anxiety alone, she should probably take an anti-anxiety medication as prescribed by a doctor. Alcohol and over-the-counter sedatives are not a wise or even effective substitute. Don't try to self-medicate or wait for feelings of anxiety to pass. Seek help now.

A Safety Net of Relationships

People with positive relationships lead more rewarding and less stressful lives that those with negative or few relationships. You are likely to have formed your positive relationships as strong ties to parents during childhood and to spouse, family, and friends during adulthood. On the other hand, losses of relationships, such as divorce, estrangement, or bereavement, reduce your sense of belonging and increase your fear of loneliness— and can have a very real and negative effect on your physical well-being. People in social isolation have been found to have higher blood pressure and other undesirable physical changes.

Your relationships form a kind of web or network, although of course not all relationships are supportive. The healthiest interactions permit you to develop as a person within familiar social settings. A social network helps you cope with stress caused by change.

Churches and Support Groups

People with religious beliefs often seem to have better health than those who don't. Many have assumed that this is because religious people tend to lead stable, low-key lives and have few health-endangering habits. But even this assumption does not explain the full extent that the studies report. A 1972 survey of more than 90,000 people found that those who attended church weekly had half the death rate from coronary artery disease of those who didn't.

I recommend participating in groups that are characterized by mutual support and in which competition is minimized, regardless of whether they are religious or secular. Local PCOSA chapters provide information from professionals, dieting help, and interaction with other women who have PCOS. Many organizations are on the Internet. The medical information may or may not be reliable, but there's no question the groups are a valuable source of emotional support.

A woman with PCOS clearly requires not only medical treatment for symptoms of infertility, irregular cycles, obesity, and skin and hair symptoms, but also help with painful psychological symptoms that strike at the heart of her identity as a woman. This should include psychological counseling and participation in PCOS self-help groups. Such counseling and group participation will go a long way in improving your quality of life and ability to cope with emotional problems.

Resources

PCOS General Information

Polycystic Ovarian Syndrome Association (PCOSA)
P.O. Box 3403
Englewood, CO 80111
http://www.pcosupport.org

This is the first public awareness group that promoted information and support for women with PCOS. It has much information on various aspects of the syndrome, and recent highlights of advances in diagnosis and treatment.

Endocrine Society
8401 Connecticut Avenue, Suite 900
Chevy Chase, MD 20815
301-941-0200
1-888-363-6274
http://www.endo-society.org

This is the site of over 11,000 clinical experts in endocrinology as well as endocrine researchers, many of whom are involved in PCOS and reproduction. Although the Web site has many endocrine subjects, a careful search of it will yield information on PCOS. A link to The Hormone Foundation, which has a major interest and involved experts in the care of women with PCOS, is provided.

The Hormone Foundation
http://www.hormone.org
For a list by state of endocrinologists expert in PCOS:
    http://www.hormone.org/resources/specialist.php3

This public education affiliate of the Endocrine Society promotes prevention, treatment, and cure of hormone-related conditions. Important handouts and fact sheets for PCOS and related hormonal conditions (e.g., obesity) can be downloaded from this site.

American Association of Clinical Endocrinologists (AACE)
1000 Riverside Avenue, Suite 205
Jacksonville, FL 32204
904-353-7878
Fax: 904-353-8185
http://www.aace.com

The AACE is an organization of over 5,000 clinical endocrinologists globally. These medical endocrinologists are board certified in endocrinology and metabolic diseases, and can be located in the medical directory. Most are qualified to treat most endocrine disorders, including PCOS. A search locates PCOS-experienced endocrinologists near your location. A search locates endocrinologists near your location. A search can also be performed for specific complaints, including PCOS, adrenal disorders, diabetes, and hirsutism, with names of specialists in these areas. Weekly news articles and guidelines for specific conditions are available, as well as articles of importance relating to PCOS.

Androgen Excess Society (AES)
http://www.androgenexcessociety.net
Contact:
Ms. Lois Dollar
Secretary to the Executive Director, Dr. Ricardo Azziz
Department of Ob-Gyn
Cedars-Sinai Medical Center
8635 West Third Street, Suite 160W
Los Angeles, CA 90048
310-423-7433
dollarl@cshs.org
FAQ with links and detailed information on PCOS:
    http://www.androgenexcessociety.org/faq.html

This group of clinicians and scientists promote knowledge of conditions such as PCOS, adrenal hyperplasia, early onset of adrenal hormone excess, and hirsutism of an undefined nature.

CARES Foundation, Inc.
866-CARES37 (866-227-3737)
http://www.caresfoundation.org

For those interested in male hormone excess in adrenal gland and associated disorders, which may mimic PCOS. Also has excellent links to many disorders.

PCOS Pavilion of ObGyn.net
http://www.obgyn.net/pcos/pcos.asp
Must-read for all.

ObGyn.net links
http://www.obgyn.net/medical.asp?page=/english/clinical
Exhaustive, with many topics of importance. Many articles feature recent data on PCOS and are written by experts.

PCOS SoulCysters
http://www.soulCysters.com

Many features and a database of articles.

PCO Teen
http://www.pcossupport.org/living/teen/about.php

A section of the PCOSA Web site, focusing on teens with PCOS.

PubMed
http://www.ncbi.nlm.nih.gov/entrez/query.fcgi

A search engine for abstracts on any topic in medicine. To look at a topic—for example, the effect of treatment of hirsutism in PCOS—enter Search as follows: PCOS and treatment and hirsutism. To learn of complications in pregnancy: PCOS pregnancy and complications. You can learn the use of PubMed via the Web sites Tutorial section. Related articles and links can be found with each citation. It is an invaluable, NIH-based source of information. Most authorities in medicine use it as a major search engine for research. Clicking on an article leads you to an abstract that may be of interest to you.

INFERTILITY

American Society for Reproductive Medicine (ASRM)
1209 Montgomery Highway
Birmingham, AL 35216-2809
205-978-5000
http://www.asrm.org

Many members, recognized leaders in this area, help answer questions relating to infertility, IVF, menopause, and other important aspects of reproductive care, diagnosis, and management. Patient fact sheets and information booklets are available, with much information on the latest in assisted reproductive technologies.

Resolve: The National Infertility Association
National Headquarters
7910 Woodmont Avenue, Suite 1350
Bethesda, MD 20814
301-652-8585
Chapter and Constituent Services
http://www.resolve.org

Provides access to all family-building options to women experiencing infertility or other reproductive disorders, along with support services, physician referrals, and education.

InterNational Council on Infertility Information Dissemination (INCIID)
703-379-9178
http://www.inciid.org

First Visit IVF
http://www.firstvisitivf.org

For those requiring information on in vitro fertilization (IVF).

The American College of Obstetricians and Gynecologists (ACOG)
http://www.acog.org

DIABETES

Council for the Advancement of Diabetes Research and Education
  (CADRE)
1250 Broadway, 36th floor
New York, NY 10001
888-771-1297
http://www.cadre-diabetes.org

Audio lectures, with slides, are presented by experts.

American Diabetes Association
http://www.diabetes.org/home.jsp

National Diabetes Information Clearinghouse (NDIC)
http://diabetes.niddk.nih.gov/

National Diabetes Education Initiative
http://www.ndei.org

Diabetes Life.Com
http://www.diabetes.com/type_2_diabetes.html

A comprehensive guide to diabetes management and insulin resistance.

WEIGHT PROBLEMS

Obesity in America
http://www.obesityinamerica.org

Latest on obesity research and treatment. There are many additional links on obesity in the Resources section. A must-read for those with obesity, whether they have PCOS or not.

American Obesity Association
http://www.obesity.org

NAASO: The Obesity Organization
http://www.naaso.org

American Board of Physician Nutrition Specialists (ABPNS)
http://www.main.uab.edu/ipnec/show.asp?durki=37725

American Heart Association
http://www.deliciousdecisions.org
Dietary guidelines and heart-healthy recipes.

American Heart Association
http://www.justmove.org
Personalized fitness recommendations, online exercise diary, and more to help
you lead a more active lifestyle.

National Institutes of Health (Obesity)
http://www.health.nih.gov/result.asp/476/29
Body mass index (BMI) calculation
http://www.cdc.gov/nccdphp/dnpa/bmi/calc-bmi.htm
http://www.asbs.org/html/bmi.html
Calculation of calories burned in various activities:
    http://www.caloriecontrol.org/exercalc.html

American Dietetic Association
http://www.eatright.org
Click on Food & Nutrition Information.

Center for Science in the Public Interest
http://www.cspinet.org

Healthatoz.com
Click on Nutrition.

Skin and Hair Problems

American Academy of Dermatology
http://www.aad.org

American Electrology Association
http://www.electrology.com

American Society for Dermatologic Surgery
www.asds-net.org/Patients/FactSheets/patients-Fact_Sheet.html

EMOTIONAL PROBLEMS

National Alliance for the Mentally Ill
24 hour/7 day NAMI Helpline: 800-950-6264
http://www.nami.org

National Mental Health Association
800-969-6642
http://www.nmha.org

American Psychiatric Association
http://www.psych.org

American Psychological Association
http://www.apa.org

National Depressive and Manic Depressive
Association (support groups in your area)
http://www.ndmda.org

National Foundation for Depressive Illness
http://www.depression.org

Anxiety Disorders Association for America
http://www.adaa.org

The Anxiety Network International
http://www.anxietynetwork.co

WOMEN'S HEALTH

American Medical Women's Association
http://www.amwa-doc.org

American Heart Association
http://www.women.americanheart.org

Web site on women's issues
http://www.ivillage.com

Microsoft Network
http://www.msn.lifestyle.com

References and Background Reading

Reference sections and bibliographies used to be only for people with special knowledge. Now, with federal funding, PubMed makes abstracts (shortened versions) of articles in most of the well-known medical journals available to everybody. To find one of the articles listed below, go to www.ncbi.nlm.nih.gov/entrez/.

Entrez is the search and retrieval system used by PubMed, and you don't have to register or be a member to find a journal article with it. You'll also find instructions on how to search for medical articles concerning keywords that you enter. PubMed was developed by the National Center for Biotechnology Information (NCBI) at the National Library of Medicine (NLM), located at the National Institutes of Health (NIH).

Following the usual practice, the titles of journals are given in abbreviated and unpunctuated form here. This is solely for convenience in keyboarding. For example, it's faster to type *JAMA* than *The Journal of the American Medical Association,* though you can get results either way.

If you would like more detailed information on something in one of the chapters, try reading abstracts about it from journals. They will probably contain some technical terms, but their overall meaning will generally be clear.

General Background References

Azziz, R., Nestler, J. E., and Dewailly, D., eds. *Androgen Excess Disorders in Women.* Philadelphia: Lippincott-Raven, 1997.

Azziz, R., Sanchez, L. A., Knochenhauer, E. S., Moran, C., Lazenby, J., Stephens, K. C., Taylor, K., and Boots, I. R. "Androgen excess in women: experience with over 1000 consecutive patients." *J Clin Endocrinol Metab* 89 (2004): 453–62.

Burrow, G. N., Duffy, T. P., and Copel, J. A., eds. *Medical Complications during Pregnancy.* Philadelphia: Elsevier Saunders, 2004.

Chang, R. J., Heindel, J. J., and Dunaif, A., eds. *Polycystic Ovary Syndrome.* New York: Marcel Dekker, 2002.

Cronin, L., Guyatt, G., Griffith, L., Wong, E., Azziz, R., Futterweit, W., Cook, D., and Dunaif, A. "Development of a health-related quality-of-life related questionnaire (PCOSQ) for women with polycystic ovary syndrome." *J Clin Endocrinol Metab* 83 (1998): 1976–87.

Dunaif, A. Polycystic Ovary Syndrome. Philadelphia: W. B. Saunders & Co., *Endocrinol Metab Clinics North Am* 28 (1999): 397–408.

Futterweit, W. "Clinical evaluation of androgen excess." In Azziz, R., Nestler, J. E., and Dewailly, D., eds. *Androgen Excess Disorders in Women.* Philadelphia: Lippincott-Raven, 1997: 625–633.

———. *Polycystic Ovarian Disease.* New York: Springer-Verlag, 1984.

———. "Polycystic ovary syndrome: clinical perspectives and management." *Obstet Gynecol Survey* 54 (1999): 403–413.

Gullo, S. *The Thin Commandments Diet.* Emmaus, Pa.: Rodale, Inc., 2005.

Redmond, G. P., ed. *Androgenic Disorders.* New York: Raven Press, 1995: 1–20.

———. "Clinical evaluation of the woman with an androgenic disorder." In *Androgenic Disorders.* New York: Raven Press, 1995; 1–20.

Speroff, L., Glass, R. H., and Kase, N. G.: *Clinical Gynecologic Endocrinology and Infertility,* 6th ed. Philadelphia: Lippincott Williams & Wilkins, 1999.

CHAPTER 1: WHAT PCOS CAN DO TO YOU

Azziz, R. "Androgen excess is the key element in polycystic ovary syndrome." *Fertil Steril* 80 (2003): 252–54.

Azziz, R., and Kashar-Miller, M. D. "Family history as a risk factor for the polycystic ovary syndrome." *J Pediatric Endocrinol Metab* 13 (2000): 1303–6.

Azziz, R., Sanchez, L. A., and Knochenhauer, E. S., et al. "Androgen excess in women: experience with over 1000 consecutive patients." *J Clin Endocrinol Metab* 89 (2004): 453–82.

Azziz, R., Woods, K. S., Reyna, R., et al. "The prevalence and features of the polycystic ovary syndrome in an unselected population." *J Clin Endocrinol Metab* 89 (2004): 2745–49.

Balen, A. H., Conway, G. S., Kaltsas, G., Techtrasak, K., Manning, P. J., West, C., and Jacobs, H. S. "Polycystic ovary syndrome: the spectrum of this disorder in 1741 patients." *Human Reproduction* 10 (1995): 2107–11.

Book, C. B., and Dunaif, A. "Selective insulin resistance in the polycystic ovary syndrome." *J Clin Endocrinol Metab* 84(9): (1999) 3110–16.

Dunaif, A. "Hyperandrogenic anovulation (PCOS): a unique disorder of insulin action associated with an increased risk of non-insulin dependent diabetes mellitus." *Am J Med* 98 (1995): 33S–39S.

———. "Insulin resistance and the polycystic ovary syndrome: mechanism and implications for pathogenesis." *Endocr Rev* 18 (1997): 774–800.

Dunaif, A., Segal, K. R., Futterweit, W., and Dobrjansky, A. "Profound peripheral insulin resistance, independent of obesity, in polycystic ovary syndrome." *Diabetes* 38 (1989): 1165–74.

Ehrmann, D. H., Barnes, R. B., and Rosenfield, R. L. "Polycystic ovary syndrome as a form of functional ovarian hyperandrogenism due to dysregulation of androgen secretion." *Endocr Rev* 16 (1995): 322–53.

Franks, S., Gharani, N., and McCarthy, M. "Candidate genes in polycystic ovary syndrome." *Hum Reprod Update* 7 (2002): 405–10.

Govind, A., Obhrai, M. S., and Clayton, R. N. "Polycystic ovaries are inherited as an autosomal dominant trait: analysis of 29 polycystic ovary and 10 control families." *J Clin Endocrinol Metab* 84 (1999): 38–43.

Kahsar-Miller, M. D., Nixon, C., Boots, L. R., Go, R. C., and Azziz, R. "Prevalence of polycystic ovary syndrome (PCOS) in first-degree relatives of patients with PCOS." *Fertil Steril* 75 (2001): 53–58.

Kaltsas, G. A., Korbonits, M., Isidori, A. M., Webb, J. A., Trainer, P. J., Monson, J. P., Besser, G. M., and Grossman, A. B. "How common are polycystic ovaries and the polycystic ovarian syndrome in women with Cushing's syndrome?" *Clin Endocrinol (Oxf)* 53 (2000): 493–500.

Marshall, J. C., and Eagleson, C. A. "Neuroendocrine aspects of polycystic ovary syndrome." *Endocrinol Metab Clin North Am* 28 (1999): 295–324.

Rosenfield, R. L., and Lucky, A. W. "Acne, hirsutism, and alopecia in adolescent girls." *Endocrinol Metab Clinics North Am* 22 (1993): 507–32.

Speiser, P. W., and White, P. C. "Congenital adrenal hyperplasia." *N Engl J Med* 349 (2003): 776–88.

Tsilchorozidou, T., Ovarton, C., and Conway, G. S. "The pathophysiology of polycystic ovary syndrome." *Clin Endocrinol (Oxf)* 60 (2002): 1–17.

CHAPTER 2: PCOS AND INSULIN RESISTANCE

AACE Insulin Resistance Syndrome Conference. Endocrine Practice. (2003): Suppl 2.

Angelico, F., Del Ben, M., Conti, S., et al. "Insulin resistance, the metabolic syndrome, and nonalcoholic liver disease." *J Clin Endocrinol Metab* 90 (2005): 1578–82.

Bray, G. A. "Risks of obesity." In Pi-Sunyer, F. X., ed. Obesity. *Endocrinol Metab Clin North Am* (2003) 32. Philadelphia: W. B. Saunders Co., pp. 787–804.

Carmina, E., and Lobo, R. A. "Use of fasting blood to assess the prevalence of insulin resistance in women with polycystic ovary syndrome." *Fertil Steril* 82 (2004): 661–65.

Dunaif, A., Segal, K. R., Futterweit, W., and Dobrjansky, A. "Profound peripheral insulin resistance, independent of obesity, in polycystic ovary syndrome." *Diabetes* 38 (1989): 1165–74.

Dunaif, A., Segal, K. R., Shelley, D. R., et al. "Evidence for distinctive and intrinsic defects in insulin action in polycystic ovary syndrome." *Diabetes* 41 (1992): 1257–66.

Dunaif, A., Xia, J., Book, C. B., et al. "Excessive insulin receptor serine phosphorylation in cultured fibroblasts and in skeletal muscle. A potential mechanism for insulin resistance in the polycystic ovary syndrome." *J Clin Invest* 96 (1995): 801–10.

Ehrmann, D. A., Barnes, R. B., Rosenfield, R. L., et al. "Prevalence of impaired glucose tolerance and diabetes in women with polycystic ovary syndrome." *Diabetes Care* 22 (1999): 141–46.

Ford, E.S., Giles, W.H., and Dietz, W.H. "Prevalence of the metabolic syndrome among US adults: findings from the third National Health and Nutrition Examination Survey." *JAMA* 287 (2002): 356–59.

Glueck, C.J., Papanna, P., Wang, P., et al. "Incidence and treatment of the metabolic syndrome in newly referred women with confirmed polycystic ovarian syndrome." *Metabolism* 52 (2003): 908–15.

Haffner, S.M., Valdez, R.A., Hazuda, H.P., et al. "Prospective analysis of the insulin-resistance syndrome (Syndrome X)." *Diabetes* 41 (1992): 715–22.

Knowler, W.C., Barrett-Connor, E., Fowler, S.E., et al. Diabetes Prevention Program Research Group. "Reduction in the incidence of type 2 diabetes mellitus with lifestyle intervention or metformin." *New Engl J Med* 346 (2002): 393–403.

Laracastro, C., et al. "Diet, insulin resistance, and obesity: zoning in on data for Atkins dieters living in South Beach." *J Clin Endocrinol Metab* 89(9) (2004): 4197–205.

Legro, R.S., Castracane, V.D., and Kauffman, R.P. "Detecting insulin resistance in polycystic ovary syndrome: purposes and pitfalls." *Obstet Gynecol Surv* 59 (2004): 141–54.

Legro, R.S., Finegood, D., and Dunaif, A. "A fasting glucose to insulin ratio is a useful measure of insulin sensitivity in women with polycystic ovary syndrome." *J Clin Endocrinol Metab* 83 (1998): 2696–98.

Legro, R.S., Kunselman, A.R., Dodson, W.C., et al. "Prevalence and predictors of risk for type 2 diabetes mellitus and impaired glucose tolerance in polycystic ovary syndrome: a prospective controlled study in 254 affected women." *J Clin Endocrinol Metab* 84 (1999): 165–69.

McFarlane, S.I., Banerji, M., and Sowers, J.R. "Insulin resistance and cardiovascular disease." *J Clin Endocrinol Metab* 86 (2001): 713–18.

Nestler, J.E. "Insulin resistance syndrome and polycystic ovary syndrome." *Endocrine Practice* 9 (Sept.–Oct. 2003): Supplement 2; 86–89.

Norman, R.J., Masters, L., Milner, C.R., et al. "Relative risk of conversion from normoglycemia to impaired glucose tolerance or non-insulin dependent diabetes mellitus in polycystic ovarian syndrome." *Human Reprod* 16 (2001): 1995–98.

Palmert, M.R., Gordon, C.M., Kartashov, A.L., et al. "Screening for abnormal glucose tolerance in adolescents with polycystic ovary syndrome." *J Clin Endocrinol Metab* 87 (2002): 1017–23.

Peppard, H.R., Marfori, J., Iuorno, M.J., and Nestler, J.E. "Prevalence of polycystic ovary syndrome among premenopausal women with type 2 diabetes." *Diabetes Care* 24 (2001): 1050–52.

Reaven, G.M. Banting Lecture 1988. "Role of insulin resistance in human disease." *Diabetes* 37 (1998): 1595–607.

———. "Role of insulin resistance in the pathophysiology of non-insulin dependent diabetes mellitus." *Diabetes Metab Rev* 9 (1993): (Suppl 1) 5S–12S.

Rosenfield, R.L. "Polycystic ovary syndrome and insulin-resistant hyperinsulinemia." *J Am Acad Dermatol* 45 (2001): (Suppl 3) S95–104.

Solomon, C.G., Hu, F.B., Dunaif, A., et al. "Long or highly irregular menstrual cycles as a marker for risk of type 2 diabetes mellitus." *JAMA* 286 (2001): 2421–26.

CHAPTER 3: PCOS AND IRS, AND
CHAPTER 4: A TANGLED WEB

Alexander, C. M., Landsman, P. B., Teutsch, S. M., et al. "NCEP-defined metabolic syndrome, diabetes and prevalence of coronary heart disease among NHANES III participants age 50 years and older." *Diabetes* 52 (2003): 1210–14.

American Association of Clinical Endocrinologists Position Statement on Metabolic and Cardiovascular Consequences of Polycystic Ovary Syndrome. Cobin, R. H., Futterweit, W., Nestler, J. H., Reaven, G. M., Jellinger, P. S., Handelsman, Y., Redmond, G. P., and Thatcher, S. S. *Endocrine Practice,* 2005.

American College of Endocrinology Consensus Statement on Guidelines for Glycemic Control. *Endocrine Prac* 8 (2002): 5–11.

Atiomo, W. U., El-Mahdi, E., and Hardiman, P. "Familial associations in women with polycystic ovary syndrome." *Fertil Steril* 80 (2003): 143–45.

Azen, S. P., Peters, R. K., and Berkowitz, K. "TRIPOD: Troglitazone in the prevention of diabetes: a randomized, placebo-controlled trial of troglitazone in women with prior gestational diabetes mellitus." *Contrl Clin Trials* 19(2) (1998): 217–31.

Baillargeon, J. P., Jakubowicz, D. J., Iuorno, M. J., Jakubowicz, S., and Nestler, J. E. "Effects of metformin and rosiglitazone, alone and in combination, in non-obese women with polycystic ovary syndrome and normal indices of insulin sensitivity." *Fertil Steril* 82 (2004): 893–902.

Balen, A. "Polycystic ovary syndrome and cancer." *Hum Reprod Update* 7 (2001): 522–25.

Belli, S. H., Graffigna, F. N., Oneto, A., Otero, B., Schurman, L., and Levalle, O. A. "Effect of Rosiglitazone on insulin resistance, growth factors, and reproductive disturbances in women with polycystic ovary syndrome." *Fertil Steril* 81 (2004): 624–29.

Birdsall, M. A., Farquhar, C. M., and White, H. D. "Association between polycystic ovaries and coronary heart disease risk in women having cardiac catheterization." *Ann Intern Med* 126 (1997): 32–35.

Boulman, N., Levy, Y., Leiba, R., et al. "Increased C-reactive protein levels in the polycystic ovary syndrome: a marker of cardiovascular disease." *J Clin Endocrinol Metab* 89(5): (2004): 2160–64.

Christian, R. C., Dumesic, D. A., Behrenbeck, T., Oberg, A. L., Sheedy, P. F., 2nd, and Fitzpatrick, L. A. "Prevalence and predictors of coronary artery calcification in women with polycystic ovary syndrome." *J Clin Endocrinol Metab* 88 (2003): 2562–68.

Cibula, D., Cifkova, R., Fanta, M., et al. "Increased risk of non-insulin dependent diabetes mellitus, arterial hypertension and coronary heart disease in perimenopausal women with a history of the polycystic ovary syndrome." *Hum Reprod* 15 (2000): 785–89.

Conway, G. S., Agrawal, R., Betteridge, D. J., and Jacobs, H. S. "Risk factors for coronary artery disease in lean and obese women with the polycystic ovary syndrome." *Clin Endocrinol (Oxf)* 37 (1992): 119–25.

Dahlgren, E., Janson, P. O., Johansson, S., et al. "Polycystic ovary syndrome and risk for myocardial infarction. Evaluated from a risk factor model based on a prospective population study of women." *Acta Obstet Gynecol Scand* 71 (1992): 599–604.

Dahlgren, E., Johansson, S., Lindstedt, G., et al. "Women with polycystic ovary syndrome wedge resected in 1956 to 1965: a long-term follow-up focusing on natural history and circulating hormones." *Fertil Steril* 57 (1992): 505–13.

Dejager, S., Pichard, C., Giral, P., et al. "Smaller LDL particle size in women with polycystic ovary syndrome compared to controls." *Clin Endocrinol (Oxf)* 54 (2001): 455–62.

Diamanti-Kandarakis, E., Houli, C., Alexandraki, K., and Spina, G. "Failure of mathematical indices to accurately assess insulin resistance in lean, over-weight, or obese women with polycystic ovary syndrome." *J Clin Endocrinol Metab* 89 (2004): 1273–76.

Diamanti-Kandarakis, E., Spina, G., Kouli, C., and Migdalis, I. "Increased endothelin-1 levels in women with polycystic ovary syndrome and the bene-ficial effect of metformin therapy." *J Clin Endocrinol Metab* 86 (2001): 4666–73.

Dunaif, A., and Finegood, D. T. "B-cell dysfunction independent of obesity and glucose intolerance in the polycystic ovary syndrome." *J Clin Endocrinol Metab* 81 (1996): 942–47.

Dunaif, A., Segal, K. R., Futterweit, W., and Dobrjansky, A. "Profound periph-eral insulin resistance, independent of obesity, in polycystic ovary syn-drome." *Diabetes* 38(9): (1989) 1165–74.

Ehrmann, D. A., Schneider, D. J., Sobel, B. E., et al. "Troglitazone improved defects in insulin action, insulin secretion, ovarian steroidogenesis, and fib-rinolysis in women with polycystic ovary syndrome." *J Clin Endocrinol Metab* 82 (1997): 2108–16.

Elliot, J. L., Hosford, S. L., Demoupolus, R. I., Perloe, M., and Sills, E. S. "En-dometrial adenocarcinoma and polycystic ovary syndrome: risk factors, management, and prognosis." *South Med J* 94 (2001): 529–31.

Elting, M. W., Korsen, T. J., Bezemer, P. D., and Schoemaker, J. "Prevalence of diabetes mellitus, hypertension and cardiac complaints in a follow-up study of a Dutch PCOS population." *Hum Reprod* 16 (2001): 5556–60.

Escobedo, L. G., Lee, N. C., Peterson, H. B., et al. "Infertility-associated en-dometrial cancer risk may be limited to specific subgroups of infertile women." *Obstet Gynecol* 77 (1991): 124–28.

Executive summary of the third report of the National Cholesterol Education Program (NCEP) expert panel on detection, evaluation, and treatment of high blood cholesterol in adults (Adult Treatment Panel III). *JAMA* 285 (2002): 2486–97.

Gammon, M. D., and Thompson, W. D. "Polycystic ovaries and the risk of breast cancer." *Am J Epidemiol* 134 (1991): 818–24.

Glueck, C. J., Papanna, P., Wang, P., et al. "Incidence and treatment of the metabolic syndrome in newly referred women with confirmed polycystic ovarian syndrome." *Metabolism* 52 (2003): 908–15.

Gu, K., Cowie, C. C., and Harris, M. I. "Diabetes and decline in heart disease mortality in US adults." *JAMA* 281 (1999): 1291–97.

Hasegawa, I., Murakawa, H., Suzuki, M., Yamamoto, Y., Kurabayshi, T., and Tnaka, K. "Effect of troglitazone on endocrine and ovulatory performance in women with insulin resistance-related polycystic ovary syndrome." *Fertil Steril* 71 (1999): 323–27.

Holte J., Gennarelli, G., Berne, G., et al. "Elevated ambulatory day-time blood pressure in women with polycystic ovary syndrome: a sign of a prehypertensive state?" *Human Reproduction* 11 (1996): 23–28.

Isojarvi, J. I., Laatikainen, T. J., Knip, M., et al. "Polycystic ovaries and hyperandrogenism in women taking valproate for epilepsy." *N Engl J Med* 329 (1993): 1383–88.

Kelly, C. C. J., Lyall, H., Petrie, J. R., et al. "Low grade chronic inflammation in women with polycystic ovarian syndrome." *J Clin Endocrinol Metab* 86 (2001): 2453–55.

Kelly, C. J. G., Speirs, S., Gould, G. W., et al. "Altered vascular function in young women with polycystic ovary syndrome." *J Clin Endocrinol Metab* 87 (2002): 742–46.

Knowler, W. C., Barrett-Connor, E., and Fowler, S. E. "Reduction in incidence of type 2 diabetes with lifestyle intervention or metformin." *N Engl J Med* 346 (2002): 393–403.

Legro, R. S., Kunselman, A. R., and Dunaif, A. "Prevalence and predictors of dyslipidemia in women with polycystic ovary syndrome." *Am J Med* 111 (2001): 607–13.

McLaughlin, T., Abbasi, F., Cheal, K., Chu, J., Lamendola, C., and Reaven, G. "Use of metabolic markers to identify overweight individuals who are insulin resistant." *Ann Int Med* 139 (2003): 802–9.

Mak, K. H., and Haffner, S. M. "Diabetes abolishes the gender gap in coronary heart disease." *Eur Heart J* 24 (2003): 1406–13.

Mather, K. J., Kwan, P., and Corenblum, B. "Hyperinsulinemia in polycystic ovary syndrome correlated with increased cardiovascular risk independent of obesity." *Fertil Steril* 73 (2000): 150–56.

Nestler, J. E. "Polycystic ovarian syndrome: metabolic and cardiovascular complications." In Kreisberg, R. A. Program Director. *Clinical Endocrinology Update 2003 Syllabus*. Miami Beach, Fla. October 24–27, 2003. The Endocrine Society Press. Chevy Chase, Md., pp. 299–303.

Nestler, J. E., and Jakubowicz, D. J. "Lean women with polycystic ovary syndrome respond to insulin reduction with decreases in ovarian 450c17 alpha activity and serum androgens." *J Clin Endocrinol Metab* 82 (1997): 4075–79.

Nestler, J. E., Stovall, D., Akhter, N., Iuomo, M. J., and Jakubowicz, D. J. "Strategies for the use of insulin-sensitizing drugs to treat infertility in women with polycystic ovary syndrome." *Fertil Steril* 77 (2002): 209–15.

Orio F., Palomba, S., Spinelli, L., et al. "Early impairment of endothelial structure and function in young normal-weight women with polycystic ovary syndrome." *J Clin Endocrinol Metab* 89 (2004): 3696–701.

Ovalle, F., and Azziz, R. "Insulin resistance, polycystic ovary syndrome, and type 2 diabetes mellitus." *Fertil Steril* 77 (2002): 1095–105.

Paradisi, G., Steinberg, H. O., Hempfling, A., et al. "Polycystic ovary syndrome is associated with endothelial dysfunction." *Circulation* 103 (2001): 1410–15.

Pierpoint, T., McKeigue, P. M., Isaacs, A. J., et al. "Mortality of women with polycystic ovary syndrome at long-term follow-up." *J Clin Epidemiol* 51 (1998): 581–86.

Polson, D. W., Adams, J., Wadsworth, J., and Franks, S. "Polycystic ovaries: a common finding in normal women." *Lancet* 1 (1988): 870–72.

Resgon, N. "The relationship between polycystic ovary syndrome and epileptic drugs: a review of the evidence." *J Clin Psychopharmacol* 24 (2004): 322–34.

Ridker, P. M. "Clinical application of C-reactive protein for cardiovascular disease: detection and prevention." *Circulation* 107 (2003): 363–69.

Segreti, E. M. "Endometrial hyperplasia and carcinoma in women with androgen excess disorders." In Azziz, R., Nestler, J. E., and DeWailly, D., eds. *Androgen Excess Disorders in Women*. Philadelphia: Lippencott-Raven Publishers, 1997; pp. 667–72.

Solomon, C. G. "The epidemiology of polycystic ovary syndrome: prevalence and associated disease risks." *Endocrinol Metab Clin North Am* 28 (1999): 247–63.

Solomon, C. G., Hu, F. B., Dunaif, A., et al. "Menstrual cycle irregularity and risk for future cardiovascular disease." *J Clin Endocrinol Metab* 87 (2002): 2013–17.

Talbott, E., Zborowski, J., and Boudreaux, M. In Daya, S., Harrison, R., and Kempers, R. *Advances in Fertility and Reproductive Medicine*. "Do women with PCOS have an increased risk of cardiovascular disease: a review of the evidence." Proceedings of the 18th World Congress on Fertility and Sterility, Montreal, Canada. May 23–28, 2004. International Congress Series, Elsevier, 1266; 2004; pp. 233–40.

Talbott, E. O., Clerici, A., Berga, S. L., et al. "Adverse lipid and coronary heart disease risk profiles in young women with polycystic ovary syndrome: results of a case control study." *J Clin Epidemiol* 51 (1998): 415–22.

Talbott, E. O., Guzick, D., Clerici, A., Berga, S., et al. "Coronary heart disease risk factor in women with polycystic ovary syndrome." *Arterioscler Thromb Vasc Biol* 15 (1995): 821–26.

Talbott, E. O., Guzick, D. S., Sutton-Tyrrell, K., et al. "Evidence for an association between polycystic ovary and premature carotid atherosclerosis in middle-aged women." *Arterioscl Thromb Vasc Biol* 20 (2000): 2414–21.

Talbott, E., Zborowski, J. V., McHugh-Pemu, K., et al. "Metabolic cardiovascular syndrome and its relationship to coronary calcification in women with polycystic ovarian syndrome." 3rd International Workshop on Insulin Resistance, New Orleans, La. February 17–19, 2003.

Talbott, E. O., Zborowski, J. V., and Boudreaux, M. Y. "Do women with polycystic ovary syndrome have an increased risk of cardiovascular disease? Review of the evidence." *Minerva Gineco* 56 (2004): 27–39.

Unique concerns for women and girls with epilepsy. http://healthology.healing well.com.

Wild, R. A., Grubb, B., Hartz, A., et al. "Clinical signs of androgen excess as risk factors for coronary artery disease." *Fertil Steril* 54 (1990): 255–59.

Wild, R. A., Painter, P. C., Coulson, P. B., et al. "Lipoprotein lipid concentration and cardiovascular risk in women with polycystic ovary syndrome." *J Clin Endocrinol Metab* 61 (1985): 946–51.

Wild, S., Pierpoint, T., Jacobs, H., and McKeigue, P. "Long-term consequences of polycystic ovary syndrome: results of a 31-year follow-up study." *Human Fertil (Camb)* 3 (2000): 101–5.

Wild, S., Pierpoint, T., McKeigue, P., and Jacobs, H., "Cardiovascular disease in women with polycystic ovary syndrome at long-term follow-up: a retrospective study." *Clin Endocrinol (Oxf)* 52 (2000): 595–600.

Chapter 5: Getting a Diagnosis

AACE Task Force Position Statement on the Insulin Resistance Syndrome. *Endocrine Practice* 9 (2003): 40–52.

Azziz, R., Carmina, E., and Sawaya, M. E. "Idiopathic hirsutism." *Endocr Rev* 21 (2000): 347–62.

Azziz, R., Sanchez, L. A., Knochenhauer, E. S., et al. "Androgen excess in women: experience with over 1000 consecutive patients." *J Clin Endocrinol Metab* 89 (2004): 453–62.

Azziz, R., Woods, K. S., Reyna, R., Key, T. J., et al. "The prevalence and features of the polycystic ovary syndrome in an unselected population." *J Clin Endocrinol Metab* 89 (2004): 2745–49.

Carmina, E. "Genetic and environmental aspects of polycystic ovary syndrome." *J Endocrinol Invest* 26 (2003): 1151–56.

Carmina, E., and Lobo, R. A. "Polycystic ovaries in hirsute women with normal menses." *Am J Med* 111 (2001): 602–6.

Chang, R. J., and Katz, S. E. "Diagnosis of polycystic ovary syndrome." In Dunaif, A., ed. *Polycystic Ovary Syndrome.* Philadelphia: W. B. Saunders Co., *Endocrinol Metab Clinics North Am* 28 (1999): 397–408.

Dunaif, A. "Current concepts in the polycystic ovary syndrome." *Annu Rev Med.* 52 (2001): 401–19.

Dunaif, A., Green, G., Phelps, R. G., Lebwohl, M., Futterweit, W., and Lewy, L. "Acanthosis nigricans, insulin action, and hyperandrogenism: clinical, histological and biochemical findings." *J Clin Endocrinol Metab* 73 (1991): 590–95.

Ferriman, D., and Gallwey, J. D. "Clinical assessment of body hair growth in women." *J Clin Endocrinol Metab* 21 (1961): 1440–47.

Futterweit, W. "Clinical evaluation of androgen excess." In *Androgen Excess Disorders in Women,* Azziz, R., Nestler, J. E., and Dewailly, D., eds. Philadelphia: Lippincott-Raven Publ, pp. 625–33, 1997.

———. "Pathophysiology of polycystic ovarian syndrome." In Redmond, G. P., ed. *Androgenic Disorders.* New York: Raven Press, 1995; pp. 77–166.

Futterweit, W., Dunaif, A., Yeh, H. C., and Kingsley, P. "The prevalence of hyperandrogenism in 109 consecutive patients with diffuse alopecia." *J Am Acad Dermatol* 19 (1988): 831–36.

Futterweit, W., Scher, J., Nunez, A. E., et al. "A case of bilateral dermoid cysts, insulin resistance, and polycystic ovarian disease: association of ovarian tumors with polycystic ovaries with review of the literature." *Mt Sinai J Med* 50 (1983): 251–55.

Goldzieher, J. W., and Green, J. A. "The polycystic ovary. I. Clinical and histologic findings." *J Clin Endocrinol Metab* 22 (1962): 325–38.

Goodman, N. F., Bledsoe, M. B., Cobin, R. H., Futterweit, W., Goldzieher, J. W., Petak, S. M., Smith, K. D., and Steinberger, E. American Association of Clinical Endocrinologists Medical Guidelines for Clinical Practice for the Diagnosis and Treatment of Hyperandrogenic Disorders. *Endocrine Practice* (2001) 7: 120–34.

Hatch, R., Rosenfield, R. L., Kin, M. H., et al. "Hirsutism: implications, etiology and management." *Am J Obstet Gynecol* 140 (1981): 815–30.

Kahsar-Miller, M. D., and Azziz, R. "The effectiveness of the interview for predicting the presence of polycystic ovary syndrome." *Gynecol Endocrinol* 17 (2003): 449–54.

Keating, N. L., Gandhi, T. K., Orav, E. J., et al. "Patient characteristics and experiences associated with trust in specialist physicians." *Arch Intern Med* 164 (2004): 1015–20.

Legro, R. S. "Polycystic ovary syndrome and cardiovascular disease: a premature association?" *Endocrine Reviews* 24 (2003): 302–12.

Lucky, A. W. "Hormonal correlates of acne and hirsutism." *Am J Med* (Suppl 1A) (1995) 89S–94S.

Moran, C., and Azziz, R. "21-hydroxylase-deficient nonclassic adrenal hyperplasia: the great pretender." *Semin Reprod Med* 21 (2003): 295–300.

Moran, C., Knochenhauer, E. S., and Azziz, R. "Non-classic adrenal hyperplasia in hyperandrogenism: a reappraisal." *J Endocrinol Invest* 21 (1998): 707–20.

New, M. "Nonclassical congenital adrenal hyperplasia and the polycystic ovarian syndrome." *Ann NY Acad Sci* 687 (1993): 193–205.

Polson, D. W., Adams, J., Wadsworth, J. and Franks, S. "Polycystic ovaries: a common finding in normal women" *Lancet* (1998) Apr. 16: 870–72.

Rosenfield, R. L. "Pilosebaceous physiology in relation to hirsutism and acne." *Clin Endocrinol Metab* 15 (1986): 341–62.

Rosenfield, R. L., and Barnes, R. B. "Menstrual disorders in adolescence." *Endocrinol Metab Clin North Am* 22 (1993): 491–505.

Rosenfield, R. L., and Lucky, A. W. "Acne, hirsutism, and alopecia in adolescent girls." *Endocrinol Metab Clin North Am* 22 (1993): 507–32.

The Rotterdam Consensus Workshop Group. Revised 2003 consensus on diagnostic criteria and long-term health risks related to polycystic ovary syndrome. *Fertil Steril* 81 (2004): 19–25.

Siegel, S., Futterweit, W., Davies, T. F., Conception, E. S., Greenberg, D. A., Villanueva, R., and Tomer, Y. "A C/T single nucleotide polymorphism at the tyrosine kinase domain of the insulin receptor gene is associated with polycystic ovary syndrome." *Fertil Steril* 78 (2002): 1240–43.

Yeh, H. C., Futterweit, W., and Thornton, J. C. "Polycystic ovarian disease: US features in 104 patients." *Radiology* 163 (1) (1987): 111–16.

Zawadski, J. K., and Dunaif, A. "Diagnostic criteria for polycystic ovary syndrome: towards a rational approach." In Dunaif, A., Givens, J. R., Haseltine, F. P., and Merriam, G. R. *Polycystic Ovary Syndrome.* Boston: Blackwell Scientific Publications, 1992; pp. 377–84.

CHAPTER 6: RIGHT FOODS, RIGHT WAY

Boschmann, M., Steiniger, J., Hille U., et al. "Water-induced thermogenesis." *J Clin Endocrinol Metabol* 88 (12) (2003): 6015–19.

Crosignani, P. G., Colombo, M., Vegetti, W., et al. "Overweight and obese anovulatory patients with polycystic ovaries: parallel improvements in anthropometric indices, ovarian physiology, and fertility rate induced by diet." *Human Reproduction* 18 (2003): 1928–32.

Food cravings: physical or emotional hunger. PharmVision.com.

Gullo, S. P. *The Thin Commandments Diet*. Emmaus, Pa.: Rodale Press, 2005.

Haiken, M. "Why can't I lose weight?" *Health* October (2004).

Harris C., and Cheung, T. *The PCOS Diet Book*. New York: Thorsons (Harper Collins), 2002.

High glycemic index foods and diabetes risk. http://www.channing.harvard .edu/nhs/newsletters/pdfs/n2002.pdf.

High glycemic index foods and heart disease. http://www.channing.harvard .edu/nhs/newsletters/pdfs/n2001.pdf.

"High glycemic index foods and increased breast cancer risk." *Environmental Nutrition*, vol. 28, no. 2 (Feb. 2005).

"High glycemic index foods and overeating." *Weil Medical College of Cornell University Food and Fitness Advisor*, vol. 7, no. 12 (Dec. 2004).

James Hill quote. http://www.washingtonpost.com/wp-dyn/articles/A63964-2005Jan10.html.

Janssen, I., Katzmarzyk, P. T., and Ross, R. "Waist circumference and not body mass index explains obesity-related health risk." *Am J Clin Nutr* 79 (2004): 379–84.

Legro, R. S. "Polycystic ovary syndrome: current and future treatment paradigms." *Am J Obstetr Gynecol* 179 (1998): 94–100.

Marano, E. H. "Chemistry and craving." *Psychology Today* Jan.–Feb. (1993).

Zemel, M. *The Calcium Key*. New York: Wiley, 2004.

CHAPTER 7: LET'S EAT

Calcium and blood pressure. http://www.ajcn.org/cgi/content/abstract/38/3/457.

Calcium and colon cancer. http://www.cancer.org/docroot/NWS/content/NWS_2_1x_Calcium_Appears_to_be_Beneficial_for_Colorectal_Cancer.asp.

Calcium and weight loss. http://www.eatright.org/Public/NutritionInformation/92_18458.cfm.

Coffee health benefits. http://www.coffeescience.org/.

Coffee health benefits. http://www.health.harvard.edu/press_releases/coffee_health_risk.htm.

The Exchange Lists for Meal Planning from the American Dietetic Association and American Diabetic Association. Revised, 1995.

Freeman, F., and Hayes, C. "Low carbohydrate food facts and fallacies." *Diabetes Spectrum* 17(3) (2004): 137–40.

Glycemic index information. http://www.diabetes.ca/Section_About/glycemic .asp.

Glycemic index of foods. http://diabetes.about.com/library/mendosagi/ngilists .htm.

Green tea and weight loss. http://my.webmd.com/content/article/22/1728_55919 .htm.

Keijzers, G. B., De Galan, B. E., Tack, C. J., and Smits, P. "Caffeine can decrease insulin sensitivity in humans." *Diabetes Care* (2) (2002) 25: 364–69.

Nuts, health benefits. http://www.nuthealth.org/cracker/nuts_show_health_benefits
.pdf.
Nuts, health benefits. http://my.webmd.com/content/article/99/105423.htm.
Omega-3 fats. http://www.americanheart.org/presenter.jhtml?identifier=4632.
Tea health benefits. http://my.webmd.com/content/article/50/40585.htm.
Tea health benefits. http://www.celestialseasonings.com/research/abouttea/
teagoodhealth.php.
Whole grains. http://www.ynhh.org/online/nutrition/advisor/whole_grains.html.

CHAPTER 8: THE PCOS EXERCISE PROGRAM

Blair, S. N., and Church, T. S. "The fitness, obesity, and health equation: is physical activity the common denominator?" *JAMA* 292 (2004): 1232–34.
"Clinical guidelines on the identification, evaluation, and treatment of overweight and obesity in adults: the evidence report." *Obes Res* 6 (Suppl 2)
(1998): 51S–209S.
Jakicik, J. M. "Exercise strategies for the obese patient." In Bray, G. A., ed. *Of-
fice Management of Obesity*. Philadelphia: Saunders, 2004, pp. 175–85.
Klein, S., et al. "Weight management through lifestyle modifications for the
prevention and management of type 2 diabetes: rationale and strategies."
Diabetes Care 27 (2004): 2067–73.
National Institutes of Health, National Heart, Lung and Blood Institute, and
North American Association for the Study of Obesity. *The Practical Guide:
Identification, Evaluation, and Treatment of Overweight and Obesity in Adults.*
Bethesda, Md.: National Institutes of Health, 2001.
Sigal, J., Kenny, G. P., Wasserman, D. H., and Castaneda-Sceppa, C. "Physi-
cal activity/exercise and type 2 diabetes." *Diabetes Care* 27 (2004):
2518–39.
U.S. Department of Health and Human Services. *Physical Activity and Health:
A Report of the Surgeon General*. Washington, D.C.: U.S. Government Print-
ing Office, 1996.
U.S. Department of Health and Human Services. *The Surgeon General's Call to
Action to Prevent and Decrease Overweight and Obesity, 2001*. Rockville, Md.:
U.S. Government Printing Office, 2001.
Weinstein, A. R., et al. "Relationship of physical activity vs body mass index
with type 2 diabetes in women." *JAMA* (10) (2004) 292: 1188–94.
Wessel, T. R., et al. "Relationship of physical fitness vs body mass index with
coronary artery disease and cardiovascular events in women." *JAMA*
292(10) (2004): 1179–87.
Wing, R. R., and Hill, J. O. "Successful weight loss maintenance." *Annu Rev
Nutr* 21 (2001): 323–41.

Chapter 9: Getting Pregnant, and
Chapter 10: Staying Pregnant

Alexander, E. K., Marqusee, E., Lawrence, J., et al. "Timing and magnitude of increases in levothyroxine requirements during pregnancy in women with hypothyroidism." *N Engl J Med* 351 (2004): 241–49.

"Assisted reproductive technology in the United States: 2000 results generated from the American Society for Reproductive Medicine/Society for Assisted Reproductive Technology Registry." *Fertil Steril* 81 (2004): 1207–20.

Baillargeon, J. P., Iuomo, M. J., and Nestler, J. A. "Insulin sensitizers for polycystic ovary syndrome." *Clin Obstet Gynecol* 46 (2003): 235–40.

Baillargeon, J. P., Jakubowicz, D. J., Iuorno, M. J., Jakubowicz, S., and Nestler, J. E. "Effects of metformin and rosiglitazone, alone and in combination, in non-obese women with polycystic ovary syndrome and normal indices of insulin sensitivity." *Fertil Steril* 82: (2004) 893–902.

Belli, S. H., Graffigna, F. N., Oneto, A., et al. "Effect of rosiglitazone on insulin resistance, growth factors, and reproductive disturbances in women with polycystic ovary syndrome." *Fertil Steril* 81 (2004): 624–29.

Bjercke, S., Dale, P. O., et al. "Impact of insulin resistance on pregnancy complications and outcome in women with polycystic ovary syndrome." *Gynecol Obstet Invest* 54 (2002): 94–98.

Bloomgarden, Z. T., Futterweit, W., and Poretsky, L. "Use of insulin-sensitizing agents in patients with polycystic ovary syndrome." *Endocr Pract* 7 (2001): 279–86.

Brettenthaler, N., De Geyter, C., Huber, P. R., and Keller, U. "Effect of the insulin sensitizer piaglitazone on insulin resistance, hyperandrogenism, and ovulatory dysfunction in women with polycystic ovary syndrome." *J Clin Endocrinol Metab* 89 (2004): 3835–40.

Elchalal, U., and Schenker, J. G. "The pathophysiology of ovarian hyperstimulation syndrome-views and ideas." *Hum Reprod* 12 (1997): 1129–37.

Fedorcsak, P., Storeng, R., Dale, P. O., et al. "Obesity is a risk factor for early pregnancy loss after IVF or ICSI." *Acta Obstet Gynecol Scand* 79 (2000): 43–48.

Futterweit, W. "Polycystic ovary syndrome: clinical perspectives and management." *Obstet Gynecol Surv* 54 (1999): 403–13.

Gerli, S., Mignosa, M., and DiRenzo, G. C. "Effects of inositol on ovarian function and metabolic factors in women with PCOS: a randomized double blind placebo-controlled trial." *Eur Rev Pharmacol Sci* 7 (2003): 151–59.

Glueck, C. J., Goldenberg, N., Wang, P., et al. "Metformin during pregnancy reduces insulin, insulin resistance, insulin secretion, weight, testosterone and gestational diabetes: prospective longitudinal assessment of women with polycystic ovary syndrome from preconception throughout pregnancy." *Hum Reprod* 19 (2004): 510–21.

Glueck, C. J., Moreira, A., Goldenberg N., et al. "Piaglitazone and metformin in obese women with polycystic ovary syndrome not optimally responsive to metformin." *Hum Reprod* 18 (2003): 1618–25.

Glueck, C. J., Phillips, H., Cameron, D., Sieve-Smith, L., et al. "Continuing metformin throughout pregnancy in women with polycystic ovary syndrome appears to safely reduce first-trimester spontaneous abortion: a pilot study." *Fertil Steril* 75 (2001): 46–52.

Glueck, C. J., Wang P., Goldenberg, N., and Sieve-Smith, L. "Pregnancy outcomes among women with polycystic ovary syndrome treated with metformin." *Hum Reprod* 17 (2002): 2858–64.

Goldzieher, J. W., and Young, R. I. "Selected aspects of polycystic ovarian disease." *Endocrinol Metab Clin North Am* 21 (1992): 141–71.

Goodman, N. F., Bledsoe, M. B., Futterweit, W., Goldzieher, J. W., Petak, S. M., Smith, K. D., Steinberger, E., Anderson, R. J., Bergman, D. A., Bloomgarden, Z. T., Dickey, R. A., Palumbo, P. I., Peters, A. L., Rettinger, H. I., Rodbard, H. W., and Rubenstein, H. A. American Association of Clinical Endocrinologists Hyperandrogenic Disorders Task Force. "Medical guidelines, for clinical practice, for clinical diagnosis and treatment of hyperandrogenic disorders." *Endocr Pract* 7 (2001): 120–34.

Hasegawa, I., Murakawa, H., Suzuki, M., Yamamoto, Y., Kurabayshi, T., and Tanaka, K. "Effect of troglitazone on endocrine and ovulatory performance in women with insulin resistance-related polycystic ovary syndrome." *Fertil Steril* 1(2) (1997) 323–27.

Jakubowicz, D. J., Iuomo, M. J., Jakubowicz, S., Roberts, K. A., and Nestler, J. A. "Effects of metformin on early pregnancy loss in the polycystic ovary syndrome." *J Clin Endocrinol Metab* 87 (2002): 524–29.

Jovanovic, L. "Glucose and insulin requirements during labor and delivery: the case for normoglycemia in pregnancies complicated by diabetes." *Endocrinol Pract* Suppl 2 (2004): 40–50.

———. "Screening and diagnosis of gestational diabetes mellitus." *Up to Date* (2004): 1–8. www.uptodate.com.

Kashyap, S., and Claman, P. "Obstetric outcome in women with polycystic ovaries" (letter). *Hum Reprod* 16 (2001): 1537.

———. "Polycystic ovary disease and the risk of pregnancy-induced hypertension." *J Reprod Med* 45 (2000): 991–94.

Kashyap, S., Wells, G. A., and Rosenwaks, Z. "Insulin-sensitizing agents as primary therapy for patients with polycystic ovarian syndrome." *Human Reproduction* 19 (2004): 2474–83.

Kenshole, A. B. "Diabetes and pregnancy." In Burrow, G. N., Duffy, T. P., and Copel, J. A., eds. *Medical Complications during Pregnancy*. Philadelphia: Elsevier Saunders, 2004; pp. 15–42.

Kinkhabwala, S., Schiano, T. D., Futterweit, W., Gambarin-Gelwan, M., Bodian, C., and Yeh, H. C. "Prevalence of non-alcoholic fatty liver disease in polycystic ovary syndrome." Abstract. Endocrine Society 87th Annual Meeting, San Diego, Calif., June 5, 2005.

Kocak, M., Caliskan, E., Simsir, E., and Haberal, A. "Metformin therapy improves ovulatory rates, cervical scores, and pregnancy rates in clomiphene citrate-resistant women with polycystic ovary syndrome." *Fertil Steril* 77 (2002): 101–6.

Kuohung, W., and Barbarieri, R. L. "Etiology and evaluation of female infertility." *Up to Date* vol. 12, no. 3 (2004): 1–10. www.uptodate.com.

Lanzone, A., Caruso, A., DiSimone, N., et al. "Polycystic ovary disease: A risk factor for gestational diabetes?" *J Reprod Med* 40 (1995): 312.

Liddell, H. S., Sowden, K., and Farquhar, C. M. "Recurrent miscarriage: screening for polycystic ovaries and subsequent pregnancy outcome." *Aust N Z J Obstet Gynaecol* 37 (1997): 402–6.

McLamrock, H. D., and Adashi, E. Y. "Pregnancy-related androgen excess." In Azziz, R., Nestler, J. E., and DeWailly, D., eds. *Androgen Excess Disorders in Women.* Philadelphia: Lippencott-Raven Publishers, 1997, pp. 601–12.

Mikola, M., Hiilesman, V., Halttunen, M., et al. "Obstetric outcome in women with polycystic ovary syndrome." *Hum Reprod* 16 (2001): 226–29.

Nestler, J. E. "Should patients with polycystic ovary syndrome be treated with metformin? An enthusiastic endorsement." *Hum Reprod* 17 (2002): 1950–53.

Nestler, J. E., and Jakubowicz, D. J., "Lean women with polycystic ovary syndrome respond to insulin reduction with decreases in ovarian 450c17 alpha activity and serum androgens." *J Clin Endocrinol Metab* 82 (1997): 4075–79.

Nestler, J. E., Jakubowicz, D. J., Evans, W. S., and Pasquali, R. "Effect of metformin on spontaneous and clomiphene-induced ovulation in the polycystic ovary syndrome." *N Engl J Med* 33 (1998): 1876–80.

Nestler, J. E., Stovall, D., Akhter, N., Iuomo, M. J., and Jakubowicz, D. J. "Strategies for the use of insulin-sensitizing drugs to treat infertility in women with polycystic ovary syndrome." *Fertil Steril* 77 (2002): 209–15.

Okon, M. A., Laird, S. M., Tuckerman, E. M., and Li, T. C. "Serum androgen levels in women who have recurrent miscarriages and their correlation with markers of endometrial function." *Fertil Steril* 69 (1998): 682–90.

Paulson, R. "In vitro fertilization." *Up to Date* vol. 12, no. 3 (2004): 1–7.

Urman, B., Sarac, E., Dogan, L., et al. "Pregnancy in infertile PCOS patients: complications and outcome." *J Reprod Med* 42 (1997): 501–5.

Vandermolen, D. T., Ratts, V. S., Evans, W. S., Stovall, D. W., Kauma, S. W., and Nestler, J. E. "Metformin increases the ovulatory rate and pregnancy rate from clomiphene citrate in patients with polycystic ovary syndrome who are resistant to clomiphene citrate alone." *Fertil Steril* 75 (2001): 310–15.

WHO Technical Support Series. Recent Advances in Medically Assisted Conception. Number 820, 1992, 1–111.

Zinaman, M. J., Clegg, E. D., Brown, C. C., O'Connor, J., and Selevan, S. G. "Estimates of human fertility and pregnancy loss." *Fertil Steril* 79 (2003): 503–9.

CHAPTER 11: SAVING YOUR SKIN AND HAIR FROM PCOS

American Association of Clinical Endocrinologists Medical Guidelines for Clinical Practice. Hyperandrogenic Disorders Task Force. Bledsoe, M. B., Cobin, R. H., Futterweit, W., Goldzieher, J. W., Petak, S. M., Smith, K. D., and Steinberger, E. *Endocrine Practice* 7 (2001): 121–34.

Azziz, R. "The hyperandrogenic-insulin-resistant acanthosis nigricans syndrome: therapeutic response." *Fertil Steril* 61 (1994): 570–72.

Azziz, R., Ehrmann, D., Legro, R. S., et al. "Troglitazone improves ovulation and hirsutism in the polycystic ovary syndrome: a multicenter, double blind, placebo-controlled trial." *J Clin Endocrinol Metab* 86 (2001): 1626–32.

Azziz, R., and Gay, F. "The treatment of hyperandrogenism with oral contraceptives." *Semin Reprod Endocrinol* 7 (1989): 246–54.

Beigi, A., Sobhi, A., and Zarrinkoub, F. "Finasteride versus cyproterone acetate-estrogen regimens in the treatment of hirsutism." *Int J Gynaecol Obstet* 87 (2004): 29–33.

Burkman, R. T., Jr. "The role of oral contraceptives in the treatment of hyperandrogenic disorders." *Am J Med* 98 (1995): (Suppl 5A), 130S–36S.

Cusan, L., Dupont, A., Gomez, J. L., et al. "Comparison of flutamide and spironolactone in the treatment of hirsutism." *Fertil Steril* 61 (1994): 281–87.

Fruzetti, F. "Treatment of hirsutism." In Azziz, R., Nestler, J. E., and Dewailly, D., eds. *Androgen Excess Disorders in Women*. Philadelphia: Lippincott-Raven Publishers, 1997, 787–97.

Futterweit, W., Dunaif, A., Yeh, H. C., and Kingley, P. "The prevalence of hyperandrogenism in 109 consecutive female patients with diffuse alopecia." *J Am Acad Dermatol* 19 (1988): 831–36.

Kelly, C. J., and Gordon, D. "The effect of metformin on hirsutism in polycystic ovary syndrome." *Eur J Endocrinol* 147 (2002): 217–21.

Lucky, A. "Hormonal correlates of acne and hirsutism." *Am J Med* 98 (1995): (Suppl 1A), 89S–94S.

Nestler, J. E., and Jakubowicz, D. J. "Lean women with polycystic ovary syndrome respond to insulin reduction with decreases in ovarian P450c17 alpha activity and serum androgens." *J Clin Endocrinol Metab* 82 (1997): 4057–79.

Pazoz, F., Escobar-Morreale, H. F., and Balsa, J. "Prospective randomized study comparing the long-acting gonadotropin-releasing hormone agonist triptorelin, flutamide, and cyproterone acetate with an oral contraceptive, in the treatment of hirsutism." *Fertil Steril* 71 (1999): 122–28.

Practice Committee of the American Society for Reproductive Medicine. "The evaluation and treatment of androgen excess." *Fertil Steril* 82 (2004): (Suppl 1), S173–80.

Redmond, G. P. "Treatment of androgenic disorders." In Redmond, G. P., ed. *Androgenic Disorders*. New York: Raven Press, 1995, 279–99.

Slayden, S. M., and Azziz, R. "The role of androgen excess in acne." In Azziz, R., Nestler, J. E., and Dewailly D., eds. *Androgen Excess Disorders in Women*. Philadelphia: Lippencott-Raven, 1997, 131–40.

Souter I, Sanchez, L. A., Perez, M., Bartolucci, A. A., and Azziz, R. "The prevalence of androgen excess among patients with minimal unwanted hair growth." *Am J Obstet Gynecol* 191 (2004): 1914–20.

Speroff, I., Glass, R. H., and Kase, N. G. *Clinical Gynecologic Endocrinology and Infertility*, 6th ed. Philadelphia: Lippincott Williams & Wilkins, 1999, pp. 1097–148.

Tartagni, M, Schonauer, M. M., Cicinelli, E., et al. "Intermittent low-dose finasteride is as effective as daily administration for the treatment of hirsute women." *Fertil Steril* 82 (2004): 752–55.

Waldorf, H. A. "Optimizing laser hair removal." *Cosmetic Dermatol* 15 (2002): 53–57.

WHO Technical Support Series. Recent Advances in Medically Assisted Conception. Number 820. 1992, 1–111.

Wong, I. L., Morris, R. S., Chang, L., et al. "A prospective randomized trial comparing finasteride to spironolactone in the treatment of hirsute women." *J Clin Endocrinol Metab* 80 (1995): 233–38.

Yemisci, A., Gorgulu, A., and Piskin, S. "Effects and side-effects of spironolactone therapy in women with acne." *J Eur Acad Dermatol Venereol* 19 (2005): 163–66.

Zinaman, M. J., Clegg, E. D., Brown, C. C., O'Connor, J., and Clegg, E. D. "Estimates of human fertility and pregnancy loss." *Fertil Steril* 65 (1996): 503–9.

CHAPTER 12: THE EMOTIONAL IMPACT OF PCOS

Bart, J. H., Catalan, J., Cherry, C. A., and Day, A. "Psychological morbidity in women referred for the treatment of hirsutism." *J Psychosomatic Res* 37 (1993): 615–19.

Brown, A. J. "Depression and insulin resistance: applications to polycystic ovary syndrome." *Clin Obstet Gynecol* 47 (2004): 592–96.

Bruce-Jones, W., Zolese, G., and White, P. "Polycystic ovary syndrome and psychiatric morbidity." *J Psychosom Obstet Gynaecol* 14 (1993): 111–16.

Coffey, S., and Mason, H. "The effect of polycystic ovary syndrome on health-related quality of life." *Gynecol Endocrinol* 17 (2004): 379–86.

Cronin, L., Guyatt, G., Griffith, L., Wong, E., Azziz, R., Futterweit, W., Cook, D., and Dunaif, A. "Development of a health-related quality-of-life questionnaire (PCOSQ) for women with polycystic ovary syndrome (PCOS)." *J Clin Endocrinol Metab* 83 (1998): 1976–87.

Eggers, S., and Kirchengast, S. "The polycystic ovary syndrome: a medical condition but also an important psychosocial problem." *Coll Anthropol* 25 (2001): 673–85.

Elsenbruch, S., Hahn, S., Kowalsky, D., et al. "Quality of life, psychosocial well-being, and sexual satisfaction in women with polycystic ovary syndrome." *J Clin Endocrinol Metab* 88 (2003): 5801–7.

Forde, E. S., et al. "Social relationships and cardiovascular disease risk factors: findings from the National Health and Nutrition Examination Survey III." *Prevent Med* 30 (2000): 83–92.

Frasure-Smith, N., and Lesperance, F. "Coronary artery disease, depression and social support: only the beginning." *Eur Heart J* 21 (2000): 1043–45.

Gallo, J. J., and Coyne, J. C. "The challenge of depression in late life." *JAMA* 284 (2000): 1570–72.

Glaser, R., et al. "Stress induced modulation of the immune response to recombinant hepatitis B vaccine." *Psychosom Med* 54 (1992): 22–29.

Guyatt, G., Weaver, B., Cronin, L., Dooley, J. A., and Azziz, R. "Health-related quality of life in women with polycystic ovary syndrome, a self-administered questionnaire, was validated." *J Clin Epidemiol* 57 (2004): 1279–87.

Helminen, A., et al. "Carotid atherosclerosis in middle-aged men: relation to conjugal circumstances and social support." *Scand J Soc Med* 23 (1995): 167–72.

Himelein, M. J. "Learning to love the one you're with: PCOS and body image." In Thatcher, S. S. *PCOS: The Hidden Epidemic*. Indianapolis: Perspectives Press, 2000, pp. 163–78.

Horsten, M., et al. "Depressive symptoms and lack of social integration in relation to prognosis of CHD in middle-aged women: the Stockholm Female Coronary Risk Study." *Eur Heart J* 21 (2000): 1072–80.

Idler, E., and Kasl, F. "Religion among disabled and non-disabled persons, II: attendance at religious services as a predictor of a course of disability." *J Gerontol Ser. D Psychol Sci Soc Sci* 52 (1997): S306–16.

Institute of Medicine, Health and Behavior: The Interplay of Biological, Behavioral and Societal Influences. Washington, D.C.: National Academy Press, 2001.

Kitzinger, G., and Willmott, J. "'The thief of womanhood': women's experience of polycystic ovarian syndrome." *Soc Science Med* 54 (2002): 349–61.

Lepore, S. J., et al. "Social support lowers cardiovascular reactivity in an acute stressor." *Psychosom Med* 55 (1993): 518–24.

Rasgon, N. L., Rao, R. C., Hwang, S., et al. "Depression in women with polycystic ovary syndrome: clinical and biochemical correlates." *J Affect Disord* 74 (2003): 299–304.

Ruberman, W., et al. "Psychosocial influences on mortality after myocardial infarction." *N Engl J Med* 311 (1984): 552–59.

Sonino, N., Fava, G. A., Mani, E., Belluardo, P., and Boscaro, M. "Quality of life in hirsute women." *Postgrad Med J* 69 (1993): 186–89.

Trent, M. E., Rich, M., Austin, S. B., et al. "Quality of life in adolescent girls with polycystic ovary syndrome." *Arch Pediatr Adolesc Med* 156 (2002): 556–60.

Weiner, C. L., Primeau, M., and Ehrmann, D. A. "Androgens and mood dysfunction in women: comparison of women with polycystic ovarian syndrome to healthy controls." *Psychosom Med* 66 (2004): 356–62.

Glossary

Abdominal fat: Fat that is centrally distributed between the chest cavity and pelvis. Also known as central or visceral fat.

Acanthosis nigricans: A skin change commonly associated with excess insulin and insulin resistance. The skin in affected areas has a darker pigmentation and often has a velvety feel and raised, dark plaques. The areas most commonly affected include the back of the neck, the groin, under the breasts, and over the elbows. It is frequently associated with small skin tags in the neck and under the arms.

ACTH *see* Adrenocorticotropic hormone.

Adenoma: A benign growth in a hormone-producing gland.

Adipocyte: Fat cell.

Adrenal gland: A triangular, walnut-shaped gland that lies on top of each kidney. The gland's outer portion, the adrenal cortex, produces the major stress hormone cortisol and other hormones such as androgens, estrogens, and aldosterone. The latter is an important hormone that regulates salt and water metabolism.

Adrenal hyperplasia: The enlargement of the adrenal glands due to an inherited defect. Because of this defect, the adrenals enlarge in order to produce enough cortisol and aldosterone. Because adrenal hyperplasia can result also in the excess production of male hormones, women suffering from it are often mistakenly thought to have PCOS. Adrenal hyperplasia in adult women may be fatal due to a cortisol deficiency.

Adrenal stimulation test: This test of adrenal function, used to detect the presence of adrenal hyperplasia, involves obtaining blood before and one hour after the injection of purified ACTH. Also called ACTH stimulation test.

Adrenocorticotropic hormone (ACTH): This hormone, secreted by the pituitary gland, stimulates the adrenal glands to produce cortisol and androgens. In its purified form, it is used in the adrenal (ACTH) stimulation test.

Alopecia: The thinning or loss of scalp hair in women due to increased male hormone levels or increased sensitivity to male hormones. Also called androgenic or androgenetic alopecia.

Amenorrhea: A condition in which a woman does not have menstrual bleeding or cycles for six or more months.

Androgen: A male hormone secreted by the ovary, testis, or adrenal gland. Examples are testosterone, androstenedione, and dehydroepiandrosterone (DHEA), the latter being mainly produced by the adrenal glands. Androgens are part of the steroid family of hormones (along with cortisol and estrogens). Both men and women produce them, although men produce significantly more than women. Androgens are responsible for producing many of the physical traits we consider male (body hair growth, increased muscles mass, and deepening of the voice). However, androgens are also important in women since they assure healthy muscles and bones, serve as the precursor or basic hormone type necessary for the production of estrogens, and are responsible for sexual arousal.

Androstenedione: A relatively weak male hormone; in women, produced equally by the adrenal glands and ovaries.

Angina pectoris: Severe pain in the chest associated with an inadequate blood supply to the heart.

Anovulation: Absence of ovulation. Women with PCOS often have difficulty becoming pregnant because they do not ovulate regularly. Women who do not ovulate are said to be anovulatory.

Antiandrogen: A drug used to block or reduce the effect of testosterone and other androgens in those sites or organs where they exert a male hormone effect. In patients with PCOS who have acne or hirsutism, they are used to block the action of androgens on the skin. Examples of antiandrogens include spironolactone, cyproterone acetate, finasteride, and flutamide.

Aromatase: An enzyme that converts testosterone to estrogens.

ART: Assisted reproductive technologies, a group of procedures that includes intrauterine insemination and in vitro fertilization.

Atherosclerosis: The buildup of plaque containing cholesterol and lipids on the innermost lining of the walls of large and medium-sized arteries, leading to serious vascular complications such as heart attack and stroke.

Biliopancreatic diversion: One of the most complicated of the current operative procedures in obesity or bariatric surgery that sometimes involves the removal of a portion of the stomach.

Biliopancreatic diversion with duodenal switch: Bariatric surgery that restricts both food intake and the amount of calories and nutrients the body absorbs by leaving a larger portion of the stomach intact, but dividing it and the small intestine.

Blood glucose: Glucose in the bloodstream. Also known as blood sugar.

BMI *see* Body mass index.

Body mass index (BMI): An individual's weight relative to his or her height. It can be calculated by multiplying weight in pounds by 703 and dividing that number by height in inches squared.

Cardiovascular disease: A disease of the heart or major blood vessels; any abnormal condition characterized by dysfunction of the heart or blood vessels.

Computed tomography (CT): A method of examining body organs by scanning them with X-rays and using a computer to construct an image. It is called a CT scan.

Congestive heart failure: A condition marked by weakness, edema (fluid retention), and shortness of breath that is caused by the inability of the heart to maintain adequate blood circulation in peripheral tissues and lungs.

Corpus luteum: A yellowish follicle that forms when the ovarian follicle has matured and expelled the egg at mid-cycle. It secretes estrogen and progesterone into the bloodstream. If no fertilization of the egg occurs, it diminishes after the menstrual cycle starts.

Cortisol: A steroid hormone produced by the adrenal glands responsible for maintaining the ability to process blood sugar, maintain blood pressure, and react to any stress and illness.

CT *see* Computed tomography.

Cushing's syndrome: A syndrome caused by an increased production of the hormone cortisol from a tumor of the adrenal cortex or pituitary. Sometimes it is also caused by an "ectopic" source such as a malignancy of various organs. Cushing's syndrome is characterized by obesity, weakening of the muscles, violet-colored stretch marks, and possible development of hypertension and diabetes.

Cyproterone acetate: A progestin that also blocks the effect of androgens on the skin. It is very useful for the treatment of hirsutism, acne, and alopecia. A rare side effect is liver abnormality. It is available outside the United States as oral contraceptive pills (Diane-35 and Dianette-35) and as Androcur.

Dehydroepiandrosterone (DHEA): An androgen produced by the adrenal glands. It is metabolized to DHEAS.

Dehydroepiandrosterone sulfate (DHEAS): An androgen produced almost exclusively by the adrenal glands.

Diabetes: Any of several metabolic disorders marked by increased blood glucose, excessive discharge of urine, persistent thirst, and elevation of blood sugar due to deficient insulin production or action. Thus, almost all type 2 diabetics are insulin resistant.

Dysfunctional uterine bleeding: A menstrual pattern when a woman has very irregular, unpredictable, and frequently heavy vaginal bleeding. Its most frequent cause is an absence of ovulation. When not shed in regular menstrual cycles, the endometrial lining tends to thicken excessively and then bleed irregularly and heavily. Because women with PCOS do not ovulate regularly, many of them suffer from dysfunctional uterine bleeding, which can be treated in most instances with hormonal medications.

Dyslipidemia: A condition marked by abnormal concentrations of lipids or lipoproteins in the blood, including lipid levels that are either higher or lower than normal, which is often but not always a result of obesity.

Electrolysis: Medically, a method of permanently destroying individual hairs by placing a needle into the hair follicle and transmitting a small amount of galvanic electricity to destroy the base of the growing hair.

Endocrinology: The study of the hormone-secreting glands and their production of hormones, including excessive or inadequate production of hormones leading to clinical abnormalities.

Endometrium: The inside lining of the uterus.

Estradiol: The active estrogen secreted by the ovaries.

Estriol: An estrogen, which may be converted from male hormones secreted by the ovaries or adrenals.

Estrogen: A large group of female hormones, including estradiol, estrone, and estriol. In women, the ovaries are the major source of estrogens, although some estrogens are produced by the adrenal glands as well. Both men and women produce estrogens, with women producing much greater quantities than men. Estrogen is responsible for the development of female characteristics and also stimulates endometrial growth.

Estrone: A weak estrogen, often converted from precursor male hormones produced outside the ovaries or adrenals.

Fatty liver disease: Inflammation of the liver due to an abnormal accumulation of fat cells, which may lead to liver dysfunction.

Fertilization: The process whereby a sperm and an egg combine to create an embryo.

Finasteride: A drug that blocks the effect of androgens on the skin and very useful for the treatment of hirsutism. Side effects are rare, although it can cause birth defects of the external genitalia in a male infant. Brand name is Proscar.

Flutamide: A drug that blocks the effect of androgens on the skin and very useful for the treatment of hirsutism. Side effects include frequent dry skin, rare serious liver toxicity, and birth defects in male fetus. Brand name is Eulexin.

Follicle: A small sac in the ovary that contains a developing egg and makes estrogens. It appears as a spherical mass of cells that usually contain a cavity. During each menstrual cycle the ovaries produce several follicles, each with its own developing egg. Through a complex process, one of these follicles is selected to continue developing to maturity and will ultimately rupture and release its egg. These follicles are the most common cause of ovarian cysts seen on an ultrasound. Since they are the result of a monthly cycle of development, these cysts resolve spontaneously over one or two months.

Follicle-stimulating hormone (FSH): Pituitary hormone essential in the regulation of ovarian function leading to ovulation.

FSH *see* Follicle-stimulating hormone.

Galactorrhea: A milky secretion of the breasts that may occur naturally or by pressing the breasts. It may indicate an excess of prolactin.

Gastric banding: Bariatric surgery designed to limit the amount of food the stomach can hold by sectioning it off with the placement of a band near its upper end. The band creates a small pouch, which delays the emptying of food from the pouch and causes a feeling of fullness.

Gastric bypass: Bariatric surgery that combines the creation of a small stomach pouch to restrict the intake of food and construction of a bypass of the duodenum to prevent food absorption.

Gastric glands: A group of cells that produce gastric secretions or hormones for use in the stomach or elsewhere in the body.

Gestational diabetes: The occurrence of diabetes during pregnancy.

Glucose: The most common type of sugar found in the body. The hormone insulin regulates the blood level of glucose and its use by various organs, including muscles and liver.

GnRH *see* Gonadotropin-releasing hormone.

Gonadotropin: Either of the pituitary hormones' luteinizing hormone (LH) or follicle-stimulating hormone (FSH), which regulate ovarian function and facilitate ovulation. These hormones are produced commercially in a purified and concentrated form that may be injected for ovulation induction.

Gonadotropin-releasing hormone (GnRH): The hypothalamic hormone that stimulates the production of the pituitary gonadotropins LH and FSH. For ovulation to occur, GnRH has to be synchronized at a certain pulsatile rate.

Granulosa cells: A lining of cells on the periphery of the ovarian follicle. They secrete sex hormones.

HDL *see* High-density lipoprotein.

High-density lipoprotein (HDL): A blood particle composed of a combination of lipid and protein, with a high proportion of protein and a little triglyceride and cholesterol. Referred to as "good" cholesterol, it is associated with a reduced probability of developing atherosclerosis.

Hirsutism: Excess hair growth in a male pattern in women, for example on the face, chest, lower abdomen, thighs, back, and extremities. Commonly coarse, thick, and dark, this hair is usually caused by excess androgens.

Hormone: A chemical produced by one part of the body that travels to another part of the body, where it produces an effect. Hormones are responsible for regulating practically every body function. Examples include estrogens, androgens, DHEA, and cortisol.

Hyperandrogenemia: An excess amount of androgens in the blood that frequently results in hyperandrogenism and skin changes such as acne, hirsutism, and scalp hair loss.

Hyperandrogenism: The effects of excess male hormones (androgens) in women, which include acne, hirsutism, alopecia, and irregular menstrual cycles.

Hyperinsulinemia: Hyperinsulinism, that is, a high level of insulin in the blood, most frequently resulting from insulin resistance. This may cause episodes of hypoglycemia, particularly after eating a carbohydrate-rich meal.

Hypertension: Abnormally elevated blood pressure.

Hyperthyroidism: Overactive thyroid gland.

Hypertrichosis: Excessive hair growth. Many, however, use the word to refer to the excess growth of vellus (fine and soft) hairs, as opposed to hirsutism (the excessive growth of thick, dark hairs in a male pattern). Women with hypertrichosis due to the excess growth of vellus hair do not have androgen excess, as in PCOS and other male hormone excess disorders.

Hypoglycemia: A low blood sugar level. Hypoglycemic episodes are frequently observed in people with insulin resistance who consume excessive amounts of carbohydrates such as sugars or starches. The high insulin levels secreted by the pancreas after they eat sugars or starches lead to a rapid drop in the blood sugar level.

Hypothalamus: The brain gland that controls a number of body functions, including mood, appetite, sleep, and reproduction. The pituitary hormones LH and FSH are stimulated by its secretion of GnRH.

Hypothyroidism: Underactive thyroid gland. This may be caused by an inherent defect or by an abnormality of the pituitary hormonal stimulus of the thyroid gland.

Idiopathic hirsutism: A disorder in which women have hirsutism but ovulate normally with regular menstrual cycles, and who consistently show normal male hormone blood levels. They usually do not have insulin resistance and usually are not at risk of diabetes.

Infertility: Diminished fertility or inability to conceive, which can be caused by problems in either men or women. PCOS often is associated with infertility.

Insulin: A hormone produced by the beta cells of the pancreas, responsible for blood sugar regulation. Insulin regulates the metabolism of carbohydrates and fats, especially the conversion of glucose to glycogen, which lowers the blood sugar level. When not enough insulin is produced to maintain a normal blood sugar level, a person develops diabetes.

Insulin resistance: A subnormal response of blood sugar to a normal insulin level. With insulin resistance in muscle and fatty tissues, the pancreas compensates by producing more insulin to maintain a normal blood sugar level. Most people with type 2 diabetes mellitus are insulin resistant, as are many obese or pregnant people and those having cortisone treatment.

Insulin resistance syndrome: A combination of high blood pressure, high LDL, low HDL, high triglyceride, high insulin, or high blood sugar levels. Much of this is related to obesity and insulin resistance, and involves risk factors for cardiovascular disease and diabetes. Also known as the metabolic syndrome.

Insulin sensitizer: A drug that improves the action of insulin and generally results in a lowering of insulin and glucose blood levels in people with insulin resistance. Primarily used for the treatment of diabetes, such drugs are also promising treatments for PCOS. Insulin sensitizers include metformin, pioglitazone, and rosiglitazone.

Laparoscopic adjustable gastric banding: Bariatric surgery that places an inflatable band around the upper stomach to create a small gastric pouch, which limits food consumption and creates a feeling of fullness. The band can be adjusted over time to meet the individual's needs.

LDL *see* Low-density lipoprotein.

LH *see* Luteinizing hormone.

Lipids: Organic substances insoluble in water that, together with proteins and carbohydrates, make up components of living cells. They include fats, phospholipids, and related compounds.

Lipoprotein: Combination of lipid and protein.

Low-carbohydrate: A common designation of food containing less than average amounts of carbohydrates. Often termed low-carb.

Low-density lipoprotein (LDL): A blood particle composed of a combination of lipids and protein, with a moderate proportion of protein, a little triglyceride, and a high proportion of cholesterol. Known as "bad" cholesterol, it is associated with an increased likelihood of developing atherosclerosis.

Luteinizing hormone (LH): Pituitary hormone essential in the regulation of ovarian function leading to ovulation.

Magnetic resonance imaging (MRI): The use of a nuclear magnetic resonance spectrometer to produce electronic images of specific atoms and molecular structures in solids, especially human cells, tissues, and organs.

Malnutrition: A condition due to an insufficient or poorly balanced diet. This may also occur due to faulty digestion or utilization of foods, and serious illnesses.

Menstrual cycle: The period of time between the beginning of one menstrual period and the next. It usually is twenty-eight to thirty days long.

Metabolic syndrome *see* Insulin resistance syndrome.

Metabolism: The chemical processes occurring within a living cell or organism that are necessary for the maintenance of life.

MRI *see* Magnetic resonance imaging.

Obesity: Excessive amount of body fat in relation to the lean body mass, or a body weight that is 30 percent over the ideal weight for a specified height.

Oligomenorrhea: Infrequent menstrual periods, at intervals greater than thirty-five to forty days, common in women affected with PCOS.

Oral contraceptive: A pill containing a mixture of an estrogen and progestin. Because they inhibit ovulation, the pills are used to prevent pregnancy. In the treatment of PCOS, they are used to control irregular uterine bleeding arising from oligomenorrhea and to decrease androgen production by the ovaries.

Ovarian cyst: A fluid-filled, balloon-like area in the ovary. Ovarian cysts measuring about an inch are usually follicles. Larger cysts may rarely be benign tumors or even cancer.

Ovary: One of a pair of glands located in the pelvis of a woman. They produce hormones, including estrogens, androgens, and progesterone, and release an egg. They are most active hormonally during the reproductive years.

Overweight: An increased body weight between 25 and 29.9 percent over an ideal weight for a specific height, as measured by the BMI. It may not only be due to an increase in body fat, but to lean muscle as well.

Ovulation: The process of releasing an egg or ovum from the ovary. Ovulation must occur in order to achieve pregnancy.

Ovulation induction: A treatment that improves the likelihood of ovulation in women seeking to become pregnant, for example, those with PCOS. Common ovulation induction agents include clomiphene citrate (Serophene and Clomid) and menotropins or gonadotropins (Pergonal, Humegon, Repronex, Follistim, and Gonal-F).

Ovum: The medical term for the egg located in one of the ovarian follicles that is normally selected to be released during ovulation.

Pancreas: A glandular organ located in the abdomen that is responsible for the production of insulin. When the pancreas is unable to provide adequate insulin to maintain a normal blood sugar level, diabetes results.

PCOS *see* Polycystic ovary syndrome.

Pioglitazone: A thiazolidinedione drug that improves the sensitivity of the body to insulin. It is used in the treatment of diabetes and it may be a promising treatment for the insulin resistance of PCOS. The brand name is Actos.

Pituitary: A gland located at the base of the brain that is responsible for regulation of many body functions, including ovulation, adrenal function, growth function, and thyroid function. Abnormalities in the pituitary can lead to erratic ovulation. When considering the diagnosis of PCOS, it is important to exclude a pituitary abnormality that could explain the irregular periods.

Polycystic: A term that means "many cysts." Because women with PCOS do not ovulate normally, their ovaries usually contain many small follicles that have failed to ovulate. These cysts are located just below the surface (cortex) of the ovary. The presence of these ovarian cysts leads to the typical "polycystic" appearance of the ovaries in PCOS, as seen on an ultrasound examination. This appearance can also be seen in other disorders that may cause irregular or abnormal ovulation even in normal women.

Polycystic ovary syndrome (PCOS): The most common hormonal disorder in reproductive-age women associated with erratic menstrual cycles, infertility, and male-hormone-related skin changes.

Progesterone: A female hormone secreted by the ovary after ovulation. It creates an environment within the uterus that is receptive to a developing embryo. Progesterone also protects the endometrium from abnormal buildup and development of cancer.

Progestin: A synthetic progesterone-like hormone.

Prolactin: A pituitary hormone that, when produced in excess (hyperprolactinemia), can result in irregular or infrequent ovulation. It should be excluded as a cause before PCOS is diagnosed.

Receptor: A protein molecule on the surface or within a cell that binds to a specific factor, such as a hormone, drug, or antigen.

Rosiglitazone: A thiazolidinedione drug that improves the sensitivity of the body to insulin. It is used in the treatment of diabetes and is a promising treatment for the insulin resistance of PCOS. The brand name is Avandia.

Roux-en-Y gastric bypass: Bariatric surgery that reduces the size of the stomach and causes poor absorption of calories, vitamins, and minerals. This procedure creates a pouch out of a small portion of the stomach and attaches it directly to the small intestine, bypassing a large part of the stomach and duodenum, or the initial portion of the small intestine.

Sedentary: Having little activity or exercise as a way of life.

Sleep apnea: A temporary suspension of breathing that occurs repeatedly during sleep, often affecting overweight people. It is a potentially serious condition, which may also be caused by a respiratory obstruction, an abnormally small throat opening, or a neurological disorder.

Spironolactone: A relatively mild diuretic (a drug that increases one's ability to urinate and lose water from the body), it has the capacity to block the effect of androgens on the skin. It is very useful for the treatment of hirsutism. Side effects include frequent urination, excess thirst, low blood pressure, feeling tired or faint, dry skin, mood disturbances, reduced libido, and heartburn. It can also cause external genital birth defects in a male infant if used during pregnancy. The brand name is Aldactone.

Sterility: A complete inability to become pregnant. Although sometimes used to mean infertility, sterility generally suggests a more permanent inability to become pregnant, such as having one's tubes tied.

Stroke: A blockage or rupture of a blood vessel to the brain. This may be associated with atherosclerosis or the passage of a blood clot.

Stroma: The central portion of the ovary, containing connective tissue and cells that produce androgens.

Testosterone: A powerful male hormone produced, in women, by the ovaries and the adrenal glands.

Theca cells: A lining of cells surrounding the granulosa cells of the egg follicle. They have LH receptors and produce androgens.

Thyroid: A gland in the frontal portion of the neck that produces hormones designed to regulate the body's metabolism. Over- or underfunction of this gland creates disturbances of most major organ functions. Abnormal production of thyroid hormones can lead to irregular menstrual cycles. When evaluating a woman with irregular menstrual periods or infertility, it is important to exclude the possibility of thyroid dysfunction before diagnosing PCOS. This does not usually present a difficult problem.

Triglycerides: A type of fat found in blood and food, the most common type of fat in the body, and a major source of energy. Triglycerides commonly circulate in the blood in the form of lipoproteins.

Type 2 diabetes mellitus: The most common form of diabetes mellitus, it occurs when the pancreas cannot make sufficient insulin to compensate for insulin resistance.

Underweight: Weighing less than is normal or healthy.

Uterine: Involving the uterus, as in uterine cancer or a uterine fibroid.

Uterus: A muscular organ above the vagina whose inner lining is called the endometrium, and whose function is to carry a fetus.

Vertical banded gastroplasty: Bariatric surgery that involves construction of a small pouch in the stomach, emptying through a narrow opening into the stomach and duodenum.

Virilization: Masculine appearance of a woman due to a high excess of male hormones, with voice pitch deeper, musculature prominent, significant male pattern hair loss, significant reduction in breast size, and excessive facial and body hair. The hallmark of virilization is an enlarged clitoris (clitoromegaly). Adrenal or ovarian testosterone-secreting tumors or other rare types of androgen excess disorders may cause this condition.

Waist circumference: A measurement around the waist used to assess abdominal fat.

Acknowledgments

So many people have been an integral part of my life and work, and I will always be grateful to them. I have received the utmost support and caring from my wife, Gloria, throughout my life and I would not have been able to persevere and continue my chosen career without her. I had wonderful childhood friends, Phil Mintz, Larry Turkell, and Burton Rabinowitz, whose baseball talk all day and our street games of punchball and stickball were a joyful part of my life. Frankly, I hope I finally convinced them that Pee Wee Reese of the Dodgers was a better shortstop than Phil Rizzuto.

As I continued along the path of my career there were many who made great contributions to my development. I wish to thank my mentors, friends, and colleagues who offered me the opportunity to exchange ideas, offered encouragement, and broadened my horizons and knowledge in many spheres. Many outstanding physicians and scientists in the various medical specialties, particularly the Department of Internal Medicine of The Mount Sinai Medical Center and Mount Sinai School of Medicine (MSSM), have been a source of inspiration to me. The standards of medical excellence and integrity of the institution have been ingrained in me since my Fellowship in the Division of Endocrinology and have served me well as a clinician and teacher of medical students and endocrine fellows. My colleagues of the Endocrine Division of The Mount Sinai Medical Center have been more than friends—they are my second family. First and foremost is my longtime friend Dr. Lester J. Gabrilove, Professor of Medicine and acclaimed endocrinologist, who was my first mentor and who spent so much of his time in guiding me as I started my endocrinology training. I will always treasure his humane qualities and the role he has continued to play in my career. It was a great source of regret that I and the field of endocrinology lost a gifted and excellent researcher and the Chief of Endocrinology at the MSSM in 1986, Dr. Dorothy Krieger. She will be missed, and I valued her encouragement and friendship. I wish to thank Dr. Terry Davies, Dr. Rhoda Cobin, Dr. Donald Bergman, Dr. Alice Levine, Dr. David Sirota, Dr. Robert Segal, Dr. David Jacobs, Dr. Edward Merker, Dr. Elliot Rayfield, Dr. Jeffrey Mechanick, Dr. Yaron Tomer, Dr. Stanley Mirsky, Dr. Robert Fiedler, and others for their friendship and advice when needed. Many other fine physicians and members of various departments of the MSSM with their gifted expertise generously devoted their time to help me undertake my research projects. Among these were the Departments of Radiology and Division of Ultrasonography (Dr. H.C. Yeh); Genetics, Statistics, Pathology (Dr. L. Deligdisch); Obstetrics and Gynecology (Dr. N. Kase); and Internal Medicine (Drs. Arthur Weisenseel, A. Unger, J. Zacks, and the late Chairman of the Department of Medicine, Dr. Richard Gorlin). Their friendship and expertise will always be treasured.

For many years Dr. Joseph W. Goldzieher published the basic research on the histology and the clinical features of PCOS. His review articles, which combined and analyzed diverse views of the abnormalities found in PCOS, remain classics of clarity and thoroughness to this day. I truly consider him my friend and inspiration in helping me understand the boundless expanse of the polycystic ovary syndrome. Joining him in the preparation of the Guidelines for Diagnosis and Treatment of Hyperandrogenic Disorders (male hormone excess) for the American Association of Clinical Endocrinologists (AACE) was a personally rewarding experience. My association and activity in AACE has allowed me further views and interchange of ideas on the polycystic ovary syndrome, and for that I am grateful to so many of my colleagues in the organization. Of particular importance to me were the numerous meetings and interplay with the members of the Reproduction Committee and other members of AACE, which include among others Drs. Rhoda Cobin, Neil Goodman, Steven Petak, Emil Steinberger, Joseph Goldzieher, Keith Smith, Geoffrey Redmond, Paul Jellinger, Donald Bergman, and Samuel Thatcher. It should also be noted that my dear friend and colleague Dr. Rhoda Cobin, the former President of AACE, and President of the American College of Endocrinology, asked me to join her in promoting national awareness of PCOS, via the Clinical Initiatives Campaign of 2004 and 2005, to fellow endocrinologists throughout the world, to media, and particularly to women with PCOS. This was an important step in the dissemination of important data suggesting the potential of cardiovascular risks in PCOS. Ongoing AACE Awareness Conferences on PCOS and the Insulin Resistance Syndrome and their potential risks were initiated by Dr. Cobin. This led to an important meeting and press conference, which was held in Washington, D.C., September 12–13, 2005, with the co-chairmanship of Dr. John Nestler and me. This was a memorable meeting in that Dr. Nestler has been in the forefront in the treatment of many aspects of PCOS with metformin. I truly value his accomplishments and his elegance, as I do his friendship and advice.

I wish to offer my deepest gratitude to Dr. Robert Rosenfield, of the University of Chicago, for his kindness, encouragement, and friendship over the years. His wisdom and comments at meetings have been always been a source of academic clarity and thoroughness. Similarly, many members with clinical interest in PCOS in the Endocrine Society, and my colleagues in the Androgen Excess Society (AES), have been more than helpful to me, and I value their friendship and outstanding expertise in androgen dysfunction. My present close association with AES and AACE has been rewarding for a number of reasons. The interaction with these organizations has allowed me the opportunity to participate with physicians and scientists who are dedicated to important research and the dissemination of information to the women in need of direction in diagnosis and treatment of PCOS. A special thanks to my colleague and friend Dr. Ricardo Azziz, the founder of the AES, whose untiring dedication to PCOS and other male hormone excess disorders in women has played an important role in its understanding and the dissemination of such findings to other physicians and the public. There are others whom I have known as friends and as active participants in AES: Drs. Enrico Carmina, Ann Taylor, Samuel Thatcher, John Nestler, Evanthia Diamanti-Kandarakis, Richard Legro, Andrea Dunaif, Maria New, Daniela Jakubowicz, Bulent Yildiz, Renato Pasquali, Robert Norman, Onno Janssen, Sharon Oberfield, Walter Miller, Geoffrey Redmond, and others. I have the highest regard for these fine scientists and researchers who have contributed such a vast array of knowledge in the unraveling of the dysfunction, the diagnosis, and the treatment of PCOS.

My special thanks for the kind efforts and enthusiasm of Dr. Lois Jovanovic in unselfishly affording me the benefit of her vast experience in the treatment of gestational diabetes (GD) and suggestions for potential risk reduction of GD in women with PCOS. Her vast experience at the Sansum Diabetes Research Institute, in Santa Barbara, California, has been globally instrumental in helping many women with this complication of pregnancy.

As the need for facilitating information on PCOS has become an important health issue, important organizations were formed, mostly via the Internet. Most importantly the emergence of the Polycystic Ovarian Syndrome Association (PCOSA), spearheaded by Mrs. Christine DeZarn and Board of Directors, has been at the forefront for information and guidance to women with PCOS for the last ten years. It offered a role to physicians dedicated to disseminating information on PCOS to participate in local and national meetings to discuss various aspects of the syndrome to women who need guidance and information. Much credit also must be given to my friend Mrs. Barbara Nesbitt, who unselfishly devotes almost all of her time to running the OBGYN.net Web site with the PCOS Pavilion section, a storehouse of information on the polycystic ovary syndrome. She has been instrumental in helping many women with PCOS and other obstetric and gynecological disorders obtain the important latest data on their condition, and I thank her for her enthusiasm and friendship. She has amassed a virtual encyclopedia of information from a number of experts on PCOS from the OBGYN.net editorial advisors and has made it easier for women with PCOS to understand more about their condition, including the newer modalities of treatment. I also wish to mention my association with a colleague at the AES, Kelly Leight, Director of the Congenital Adrenal Hyperplasia Research, Education and Support (CARES) Foundation, for her enthusiasm in the education of those afflicted with adrenal disorders.

I wish to offer my sincerest thanks to a very special person, dear friend, and renowned colleague, Dr. Stephen P. Gullo, who has been a very special person and friend in my life. He taught me much about the role of nutrition and change of lifestyle techniques in people with weight problems. His outstanding expertise in this field, his warmth and devotion to his patients, and his contribution to the field has earned him many awards, and three interviews with Larry King on CNN. They are well earned because his books (*Thin Tastes Better* and a new one called *The Thin Commandments Diet*) are innovative classics in the world of weight control. His interest and helpful advice in the formulation and intricacies involved in the writing of this book, including almost weekly phone calls, were very instrumental in planning virtually every phase of this book. His well-known reputation as an outstanding nutritionist and weight loss expert through a proper approach to weight loss has helped many of my patients. I value his major contribution to this book, which was specially written for women with PCOS and/or the insulin resistance syndrome. It took valued time away from his patients, and I am more than honored that he did this for the noble cause of helping women with PCOS and others, many of whom have hormonal reasons for their inability to lose weight adequately.

I also am grateful for the help of an excellent and experienced nutritionist, Martha McKittrick, for her unique and helpful dietary meal planning section for women with PCOS. Many of my patients have seen Martha and are pleased with her specific suggestions for dieting and the results that they achieve. I have been delighted to know her for six years, and she graciously agrees to talk at annual as well as local chapter PCOSA meetings. Her gracious personality and knowledge was evident and noted in several mutual TV interviews on CNN and Webcasts on Healthology.com. I am grateful to her, and for the enthusiasm and professionalism of her help. She has earned a special place in my esteem of her excellent ability to make patients with PCOS follow an adequate and appropriate dietary approach. With this dream team of Stephen and Martha, I felt more than assured that women with PCOS will get the special advice on achieving and maintaining weight loss that they were looking for. Their contribution to this book is a tribute to their dedication to the art of helping those who almost feel they cannot be helped. Each of the two, Dr. Stephen Gullo and Martha McKittrick, are special to me. The long periods of time they spent in helping me with this book will not be forgotten.

My sincerest thanks go to Chase Henry Mechanick for his thorough and helpful review of several sections. My thanks also to David Nayor, who helped me with the interplay of careful communications of all involved in the dietary chapters.

I also wish to thank my friend Mrs. Molly Shulman, who graciously assisted funding my genetic research for a PCOS candidate gene at the MSSM, and who has done much to further the understanding of teens with PCOS. Her work in helping teens with PCOS has been an important strategy in getting these young teens to cope with the syndrome. I truly appreciate her kindness and also her active work with PCOSA, where she unselfishly took time away from her duties with her San Diego Padres to be so active in the organization. Another special person who has been of immeasurable help in funding my research projects is Mr. Jaqui Safra. His interest in furthering research in metabolic disorders associated with PCOS has been another reason why so much new data has emerged in the understanding of this syndrome, and the potential benefits of new approaches in its management. Ken Sawyer, a special friend and gentle person dedicated to helping women with health disorders, including PCOS, deserves my respect and thanks for his noble efforts and contributions.

My gratitude to my wonderful office staff members, who have done so much for my practice. The professionalism and hard work of Luba Dronova, Roni Malinbaum, and Richard Weiss have made my office not only pleasant and efficient but friendly and patient oriented. They are a wonderful interpersonal group who makes every patient feel special and at times makes me wonder if the patient is here to see my staff or me.

I am also grateful to Allan Noel Taffet, whose expertise was of great help to me in unraveling the technicalities and legal details relating to this book. I am forever appreciative of his sound advice and friendship.

I also have been fortunate to have the cooperation as well as valued advice of Lynn Sonberg and George Ryan. They were always receptive and helpful, and the book owes much to their time-consuming efforts. My special thanks also to Henry Holt and Company, and Sam Douglas, who oversaw the development of the book. His helpful advice and enthusiasm was much appreciated. This book was written to educate and inform the woman with polycystic ovary syndrome, thus allowing her to benefit from my experience and association with other experts over the years. In so doing, the reader will be better educated to involve herself in a careful analysis and algorithm of choices for defining appropriate treatment. To see the patient feel better, more assured, self-confident, and eventually achieve her goals in life—that was my goal and aspirations in writing this book, and I hope it was achieved. It was a labor of love, and to you my readers I wish you all the best, and a healthy and happy life. Bon voyage.

WALTER FUTTERWEIT, M.D. F.A.C.P., F.A.C.E.
Clinical Professor of Medicine (Division of Endocrinology)
Mount Sinai School of Medicine, New York, NY 10029
Co-chief of the Endocrine Clinic
Attending in Medicine
The Mount Sinai Medical Center, New York City

INDEX

urinary frequency, 182
urine microalbumin level, 68
urine protein, 175
uterine cancer, 13, 48, 53–54, 105, 180
uterine fibroids, 155
uterus, 8–9, 13, 53, 237

valproate, 25
Vaniqa (eflornithine hydrocholoride),
    186
varicose veins, 179
Vasotec. *See* enalapril
vegetables, 76, 80, 98, 104, 127,
    129
    juice, 131
    low calorie, low carb, 114–15
    opticarbs and, 133
    recipes, 135–37
virilizaton, 237
vitamin B-12, 113, 191
vitamins, 16, 89, 154
    supplements, 113

walking, 140–42, 146–48
water, 102–4, 115
waxing, 188
wedge resection biopsies, 4
weight control (loss), 74–125
    accelerated meal plans, 117–25
    artificial sweeteners and, 116
    awareness of caloric intake and,
        103
    benefits of, 28–29
    caloric needs for, 100–101
    calorie-smart options for, 104
    cinnamon and, 124
    counting calories on low-carb diet
        and, 101–3
    diabetes and heart disease and,
        52–53
    eating plan for, 111–34
    exercise and, 142–51
    fiber and, 133
    food history and, 94–99
    getting pregnant and, 153, 154
    high blood pressure and, 46

hormones and, 10
IRS and, 38, 41
low-carb diet and water loss and,
    102–4
low-fat, high-calcium dairy foods and,
    124
low-glycemic index diet for for,
    77–93
metformin and, 158–60
mood eating and, 105–10
my favorite foods and, 129–32
nuts and, 132–33
opticarbs and, 133
periods and, 12
pregnancy and, 157, 176
rapid, hair loss and, 16
recipes for, 134–38
restaurants and, 125–28
symptoms alleviated by and, xvi, xvii,
    20, 22–23, 27–28
thermogenic effects and, 127
triglyceride levels and, 41
uterine cancer and, 54
water to speed, 116
winning strategies for, 93–110
weight lifting, 151
weight problems, xiv, xvi, 5–7, 10, 71,
    139, 142, 155, 175, 194. *See also*
    overweight; obesity
    defined, 19
    hormones and, 10, 25, 63, 72
    inability to lose, 19, 33
    insulin resistance and, 26–36
    resources for, 208–9
    sleep apnea and, 21
whole grains, 80, 83, 89–90, 98
Wilmott, J., 194
women's health resources, 210

xylitol, 85

Yasmin, 179
yoga, 151
yogurt, 129–30, 133

Zetia. *See* ezetimibe

ABOUT THE AUTHOR

WALTER FUTTERWEIT, M.D., F.A.C.P., F.A.C.E., received his medical degree at the NYU School of Medicine, and did his fellowship in endocrinology at the Mount Sinai Hospital. After a year at the Worcester Foundation for Experimental Biology in Shrewsbury, Massachusetts, he returned to Mount Sinai Hospital's Division of Endocrinology and started his clinical practice in endocrinology. His research was recognized by a National Institutes of Health grant. Dr. Futterweit's interest in the polycystic ovary syndrome (PCOS) began at a time when it was considered to be a rare disease. He wrote the first textbook on PCOS, and has authored over seventy-five medical articles, twenty-five abstracts at endocrine meetings, and numerous chapters in textbooks. He lectures frequently, is co-chief of the Endocrine Clinic, and teaches at the Mount Sinai School of Medicine, where he became clinical professor of medicine in 1987. In his large practice he primarily sees women having male hormone excess problems, including almost 2,000 women with PCOS.

Dr. Futterweit has been a leader of the American Association of Clinical Endocrinologists' national campaign of public awareness of PCOS. He has also been an advocate for women with PCOS as an Advisory Board member of the Polycystic Ovarian Syndrome Association (PCOSA), where he was honored for his work over the years. His other activities include articles on PCOS for the OBGYN.net Web site. Over the last few years, much of his time has also been devoted to the Androgen Excess Society (AES) and transmission of information on PCOS through its Web site. Dr. Futterweit lives with his wife in Westchester County, New York. His three children and four grandchildren live nearby.

About the Nutrition Consultant

MARTHA MCKITTRICK, R.D., C.D.N., C.D.E., is a registered dietitian and certified diabetes educator. A staff dietitian at The New York Presbyterian Hospital for the past twenty years, she also counsels patients privately and is a consultant to physicians, corporations, and health clubs. She was nutritionist for the 1998 New York City Marathon. Ms. McKittrick has appeared on numerous television, radio, and Webcast programs. She is on the medical advisory board for PCOSA and on the editorial advisory board for the PCOS Pavilion of OBGYN.net. She is also the health expert on WebMD's Diet and Nutrition Message Board.